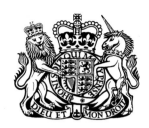

TEENAGE PREGNANCY

Presented to Parliament by the

Prime Minister

by Command of Her Majesty

June 1999

Cm 4342

£15

This report meets the Social Exclusion Unit's remit to report to the Prime Minister to:

"work with other departments, building particularly on the work already undertaken by the Department of Health to develop an integrated strategy to cut rates of teenage parenthood, particularly under-age parenthood, towards the European average, and propose better solutions to combat the risk of social exclusion for vulnerable teenage parents and their children."

The report has been prepared in consultation with all the relevant Government Departments and the Unit has been greatly helped by the many organisations and individuals who responded to its consultation exercise and arranged meetings and visits.

The Social Exclusion Unit's remit covers England only and references within the report to 'national' initiatives relate only to England. However, the analysis underlying the report, and the importance given to tackling the problem is shared by the Scottish, Welsh and Northern Ireland Offices. Together with the new devolved administrations, they will be considering whether the action set out in the report could be applied in the light of the particular circumstances present in each country.

CONTENTS

FOREWORD BY THE PRIME MINISTER

Britain has the worst record on teenage pregnancies in Europe. It is not a record in which we can take any pride. Every year some 90,000 teenagers in England become pregnant. They include nearly 8,000 who are under 16. Some of these teenagers, and some of their children, live happy and fulfilled lives. But far too many do not.

Teenage mothers are less likely to finish their education, less likely to find a good job, and more likely to end up both as single parents and bringing up their children in poverty. The children themselves run a much greater risk of poor health, and have a much higher chance of becoming teenage mothers themselves. Our failure to tackle this problem has cost the teenagers, their children and the country dear.

What is even worse is that the high rate of teenage pregnancies is not inevitable. While the rate of teenage pregnancies has remained high here, throughout most of the rest of Western Europe it fell rapidly.

As a country, we can't afford to continue to ignore this shameful record. Few societies find it easy to talk honestly about teenagers, sex and parenthood. It can seem easier to sweep such uncomfortable issues under the carpet. But the consequences of doing this can be seen all round us in shattered lives and blighted futures.

That's why I asked the Social Exclusion Unit to study the reasons for our record on teenage pregnancies, and to develop a strategy to cut the rates of teenage parenthood.

The report reveals the scale of the problem we face in this country and the cycle of despair in which many teenage parents are trapped. It also shows how too many teenage mothers – and fathers – simply fail to understand the price they, their children and society, will pay.

It sets out just how poorly informed many British children are about sex and parenthood, contraception and sexually transmitted infections. It makes clear that while more than two-thirds of young people do not have sex before their 16th birthday, too many of those who do lack the knowledge or confidence to say no, or not yet.

Let me make one point perfectly clear. I don't believe young people should have sex before they are 16. I have strong views on this. But I also know that no matter how much we might disapprove, some do. We shouldn't condone their actions. But we should be ready to help them avoid the very real risks that under-age sex brings. The fact is that unprotected sex at any age is dangerous.

But the report is not just about what has gone wrong. It sets out how we can put it right. It contains a package of measures to help dramatically reduce the rate of teenage pregancies in Britain and to tackle social exclusion among young parents and their families.

It sets out what we are doing to improve education and job opportunities. Most teenagers who are likely to become pregnant come from poor areas, and from disadvantaged backgrounds. Often they feel they have nothing to lose by becoming pregnant. They badly need help at school and support to find jobs and follow a career.

It calls for a concerted campaign, involving all the different agencies and including religious leaders and the media to give a clear and consistent message to teenagers about the real impact of pregnancy and parenthood on their lives. It shows how we can and must improve education on relationships and sex for teenagers. We must give teenagers the confidence and the information so they don't feel compelled to have sex. No one should become pregnant or contract a sexually transmitted infection because of ignorance.

It highlights, too, the importance of ensuring that teenagers are aware of the real responsibilities of being a parent, including the financial responsibilities of being a father. That means a bigger role for the Child Support Agency to ensure that all fathers, including teenage fathers, cannot simply walk away from their children.

We must also do more to support teenagers if they do have a child. They should be strongly encouraged to complete their education and keep in touch with the jobs market. Young mothers should not be isolated in flats on their own. So we want to encourage teenagers either to stay with their own parents or to move into supervised accommodation.

This is a comprehensive programme of action which we will put into practice straight away. Our ambitious goal is to halve the rate of teenage pregnancies in ten years. It will not be easy. It will mean putting aside prejudice and embarrassment to engage in a mature debate. But we owe it to today's and tomorrow's teenagers to get this right at last.

Tony Blair

SUMMARY

Scale

1. In England, there are nearly 90,000 conceptions a year to teenagers; around 7,700 to girls under 16 and 2,200 to girls aged 14 or under. Roughly three-fifths of conceptions – 56,000 – result in live births. Although more than two-thirds of under 16s do not have sex and most teenage girls reach their twenties without getting pregnant, the UK has teenage birth rates which are twice as high as in Germany, three times as high as in France and six times as high as in the Netherlands. Some other countries – notably the US – have rates even higher than the UK. But within Western Europe, the UK now stands out as having the highest rate of teenage births. This report sets out the Social Exclusion Unit's analysis of the problem; the decisions the Government has made about how to tackle it; and some issues on which the Government would welcome views.

Why it matters

2. The facts are stark:

   ■ This is a problem which affects just about every part of the country. Even the most affluent areas in England have teenage birth rates which are high by European standards.

   ■ But it is far worse in the poorest areas and among the most vulnerable young people, including those in care and those who have been excluded from school.

   ■ Although less than a third are sexually active by the time they are 16, half of those who are use no contraception the first time, with hindsight most young women wish they had waited and for a significant group, sex is forced or unwanted.

   ■ Teenagers who do not use contraception have a 90 per cent chance of conceiving in one year and those who do not use condoms are also exposed to a range of sexually transmitted infections (STIs). In a single act of unprotected sex with an infected partner, teenage women have a 1 per cent chance of acquiring HIV, a 30 per cent risk of getting genital herpes and a 50 per cent chance of contracting gonorrhoea.

   ■ Of those who do get pregnant, half of under 16s and more than a third of 16 and 17 year olds opt for abortion – that means just over 15,000 under 18s a year having an abortion.

   ■ Ninety per cent of teenage mothers have their babies outside marriage, and relationships started in the teenage years have at least a 50 per cent chance of breaking down.

   ■ Teenage parents are more likely than their peers to live in poverty and unemployment and be trapped in it through lack of education, child care and encouragement.

   ■ The death rate for the babies of teenage mothers is 60 per cent higher than for babies of older mothers and they are more likely to have low birth weights, have childhood accidents and be admitted to hospital. In the longer term, their daughters have a higher chance of becoming teenage mothers themselves.

Why are rates in the UK so high?

3.   In the 1970s, the UK had similar teenage birth rates to other European countries. But while they achieved dramatic falls in the 1980s and 1990s, the rates in the UK remained stuck.

4.   However, there is no single explanation for their relative success and the UK's relative failure; individual decisions about sex and parenthood are never simple to understand. But three factors stand out:

5.   The first is **low expectations**. Throughout the developed world, teenage pregnancy is more common amongst young people who have been disadvantaged in childhood and have poor expectations of education or the job market. One reason why the UK has such high teenage pregnancy rates is that there are more young people who see no prospect of a job and fear they will end up on benefit one way or the other. Put simply, they see no reason not to get pregnant.

6.   The second is **ignorance**. Young people lack accurate knowledge about contraception, STIs, what to expect in relationships and what it means to be a parent. Only around half of under 16s and two-thirds of 16–19s use contraception when they start to have sex, compared with around 80 per cent in the Netherlands, Denmark or the US. The reality of bringing up a child, often alone and usually on a low income, is not being brought home to teenagers and they are often quite unprepared for it. They do not know how easy it is to get pregnant and how hard it is to be a parent.

7.   The third is **mixed messages**. As one teenager put it to the Unit, it sometimes seems as if sex is compulsory but contraception is illegal. One part of the adult world bombards teenagers with sexually explicit messages and an implicit message that sexual activity is the norm. Another part, including many parents and most public institutions, is at best embarrassed and at worst silent, hoping that if sex isn't talked about, it won't happen. The net result is not less sex, but less protected sex.

8.   These three factors point to a single faultline in past attempts to tackle this problem: neglect. Governments and society have neglected the issue because it can easily drift into moralising and is difficult for anyone to solve on their own. And the most vulnerable communities and young people have been the most neglected of all. Teenage pregnancy is a classic joined-up problem but has never had an agency or individual prepared to take responsibility for tackling it as a whole.

What next?

9.   As societies and economies become ever more dependent on skills and knowledge, the personal and societal costs of allowing significant numbers of teenagers to drop out of education are much higher than they were a generation ago and in societies with far better access to information than in the past, there are no good reasons why teenagers should be as ignorant as they are about the facts of life and the role of contraception.

10. The UK cannot afford high rates of teenage conception and parenthood at the end of the 20th century. Other developed countries have seen their rates steadily fall.

11. There is now a need to do better, drawing on a clear analysis of the problem, having realistic but demanding goals and credible means of achieving them. There are many Government programmes aimed at giving young people a better start in adult life and these will help, but the specific issue of teenage pregnancy needs a specific remedy as well.

12. The Unit's analysis has highlighted two main goals:

   ■ Reducing the rate of teenage conceptions, with the specific aim of halving the rate of conceptions among under 18s by 2010.

   ■ Getting more teenage parents into education, training or employment, to reduce their risk of long term social exclusion.

Action plan

13. The action for achieving these goals falls into four categories:

   ■ **A national campaign**, involving Government, media, voluntary sector and others to improve understanding and change behaviour.

   ■ **Joined-up action** with new mechanisms to co-ordinate action at both national and local levels and ensure that the strategy is on track.

   ■ **Better prevention** of the causes of teenage pregnancy, including better education in and out of school, access to contraception, and targeting of at-risk groups, with a new focus on reaching young men, who are half of the solution, yet who have often been overlooked in past attempts to tackle this issue.

   ■ **Better support** for pregnant teenagers and teenage parents, with a new focus on returning to education with child care to help, working to a position where no under 18 lone parent is put in a lone tenancy, and pilots around the country providing intensive support for parents and child.

NATIONAL CAMPAIGN

14. **Government cannot reduce rates of teenage conception and pregnancy on its own. To achieve the goals set out above, there needs to be nothing less than a common national effort to change the culture surrounding teenage pregnancy, involving Government and professionals, opinion formers and the media, communities, parents and teenagers themselves, in sending much clearer messages about teenage sex and pregnancy.**

15. To achieve these goals:

   ■ *the national campaign will target young people and parents with the facts about teenage pregnancy and parenthood, with advice on how to deal with the pressures to have sex, and with messages that underline the importance of using contraception if they do have sex; and*

   ■ *local campaigns in areas of high teenage pregnancy will be developed in collaboration with print and broadcast media and with youth, faith and other organisations, to reinforce the message.*

JOINED-UP ACTION

16. **To maximise the impact of the various measures set out above, it will be essential to put in place new structures that co-ordinate action both nationally and locally.**

   At a national level:

   ■ *a new task force of Ministers and an implementation unit led by the Department of Health will ensure that Whitehall keeps focused on achieving the reduction in teenage parenthood rates; and*

   ■ *an independent national advisory group on teenage pregnancy will be set up to advise Government and monitor the success of the whole strategy.*

   At a local level:

   ■ *there will be an identified local co-ordinator to pull together all the local services that have a role in preventing teenage pregnancy or supporting those that become parents. The local community will be consulted and encouraged to play a part in achieving the reductions. There will be extra money from central government to help in high rate areas.*

BETTER PREVENTION

17. **To reduce the teenage pregnancy rates at all ages, young people have to be prepared far more effectively for sex and relationships, ensuring that they have the means to deal with the pressure to have sex too soon. Parents are vital to ensuring this happens, and they deserve better help in talking to their children. Young men are half of the solution, yet they have often been overlooked in education and in designing services. Groups at special risk of teenage pregnancy need special help to avoid it. Specific measures include:**

   ■ *new guidance for schools on sex and relationships education which helps young people deal with the pressures to have sex too young, and encourages them to use contraception if they do have sex;*

   ■ *new school inspection and better training for teachers to bolster the new guidance;*

   ■ *a new emphasis on consulting parents about what their children should be taught about sex and relationships, and practical help for them to talk to children about sex themselves;*

   ■ *information campaigns to explain what support is available to parents in talking about sex and relationships with their children;*

   ■ *local implementation fund for integrated and innovative programmes (including, for example, peer mentoring) in high rate areas;*

   ■ *new health service standards for effective and responsible contraceptive advice and treatment for young people;*

   ■ *clear and credible guidance for health professionals on the prescription, supply and administration of contraceptives to under 16s, including a duty to counsel them when they seek advice on contraception;*

- *a new national helpline to give advice to teenagers on sex and relationships and to direct them to local services;*

- *a national publicity campaign to tell young people they can talk to health professionals about sex and contraception in confidence;*

- *targeting young men with information about the consequences of sex and fatherhood, including the financial responsibility to support their children;*

- *sex and relationships education in and out of school will give particular attention to involving young men;*

- *getting social services to give priority to preventing teenage pregnancy for the children in their care;*

- *Young Offenders Institutions all offering parenting and sexual health classes;*

- *giving sex and relationships education to children excluded from school; and*

- *improving the overall framework for 16–18 year olds not benefiting from education, training or employment (this is the subject of the Unit's next report).*

BETTER SUPPORT

18. **Teenagers who become parents should not lose out on opportunities for the future. Young parents should have the chance to complete their education and prepare to support themselves and their family. Housing policies that have treated very young parents as if they were already adults need to be reformed. Specifically that means:**

- *better co-ordination so that pregnant teenagers get advice and support to stop them falling through the cracks;*

- *under 16 year old mothers will be required to finish their full time education, and be given help with child care to ensure this happens;*

- *16 and 17 year old parents will be able to take part in the Education Maintenance Allowance Pilots from September 1999.*

- *new help for teenage parents claiming benefit to find a job;*

- *a piloted new support package for young parents to help them with housing, health care, parenting skills, education and child care;*

- *the solution for 16 and 17 year old mothers who cannot live with parents or partner must be supervised semi-independent housing with support, not a tenancy on their own; and*

- *the Child Support Agency (CSA) will target fathers of children of under 18 year old mothers for early child support action.*

Conclusion

19. This adds up to a 10 year programme to improve the climate in which young people prepare for adulthood, and the support for teenage parents and their children. Annex 10 poses some questions for consultation on implementation mechanisms for the programme, and the Government will start work immediately on the rest of the programme. Funding of some £60 million over the next three years has already been identified. A new unit in the Department of Health which will co-ordinate the work, will be set up in the autumn of 1999. The targets are challenging, but are the minimum the Government should aim for if there is to be a lasting improvement. The success of other countries shows that high teenage conception rates are not inevitable and that they can be brought down quickly.

20. Teenage pregnancy is not an easy issue for any government to tackle. It touches on very strongly held beliefs and intimate decisions. But the costs of neglect are too high. Action on a range of fronts is now long overdue. With carefully considered and consistently implemented policies, a step change can be made that brings benefits in fewer unwanted pregnancies, fewer children brought up in poverty and successive generations of children and young people having better chances for the future.

1. TEENAGE PARENTS: SCALE AND TRENDS

> There are nearly 90,000 teenage conceptions a year in England resulting in 56,000 live births. Around 7,700 conceptions are to under 16s. This rate is higher than any other Western European country. The UK has not matched their success in reducing rates in the 1980s and 1990s. Ninety per cent of teenage births are outside marriage.

Scale

1.1 In 1997, in England:

- almost 90,000 teenagers became pregnant;

- roughly three-fifths went on to give birth, 56,000 in total;

- almost 7,700 conceptions were to under 16s (about 70 per cent to 15 year olds), resulting in 3,700 births;

- 2,200 conceptions were to girls aged 14 or under; and

- around 50 per cent of conceptions to under 16s ended in abortion.[1]

Figure 1: Teenage conceptions – outcome by age at conception, England 1997

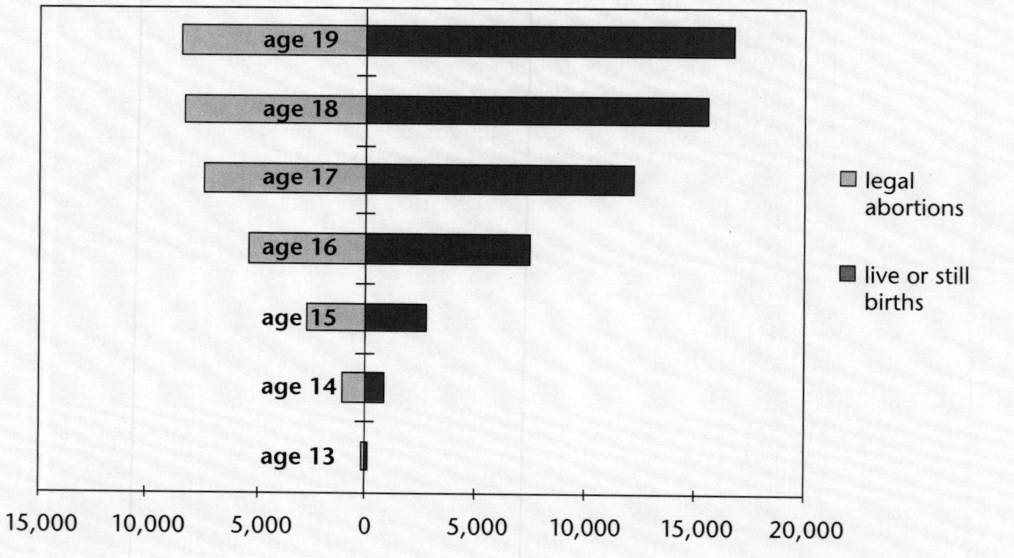

Source: ONS. Figures do not include miscarriages or illegal abortions.

1.2 A significant number of young women conceive more than once in their teens; one in six teenagers who had an abortion in 1997 had already had an abortion or a live birth, and 2 per cent had both.[2] One survey found that around one in eight young women who had their first baby in their teens went on to have a second child before they were 20.[3]

1.3 It is estimated that around 87,000 children in England today have a teenage mother.[4] Four per cent of adult men and 13 per cent of adult women report having had a child under 20.[5] The difference is explained by the fact that partners of teenage mothers are typically between 3.5 and 5 years older than them.[6]

International comparisons

1.4 **Figure 2** shows that the UK has the highest rate of teenage births in Western Europe; twice that in Germany, three times that in France and six times the Dutch rate. The UK is nearer to the rates in other English speaking countries, and the US and New Zealand rates are much higher.

1.5 The UK's ratio of teenage abortions is higher than in some comparable countries and lower than others. See **Figure 16** in Chapter 4.

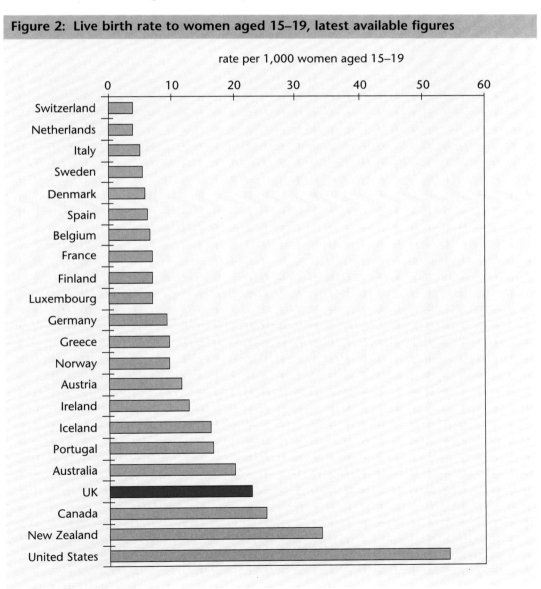

Figure 2: Live birth rate to women aged 15–19, latest available figures

rate per 1,000 women aged 15–19

Source: Eurostat & Centre for Sexual Health Research, Southampton (Annex 1 refers).

The UK

1.6 Rates within the UK vary between the different countries. Scotland, Northern Ireland and England have teenage birth rates of around 30 per 1,000 women. Wales is higher with a teenage birth rate of 37.7 per 1,000; this is similar to some areas in England.

Trends

1.7 Throughout most of Western Europe, teenage birth rates fell during the 1970s, 1980s and 1990s, but the UK rates have been stuck at the early 1980s level or above. **Figure 3** illustrates this, and **Figure 4** shows trends for the English speaking countries.

Figure 3: Live birth rate to women aged 15–19: various European countries 1973–1996

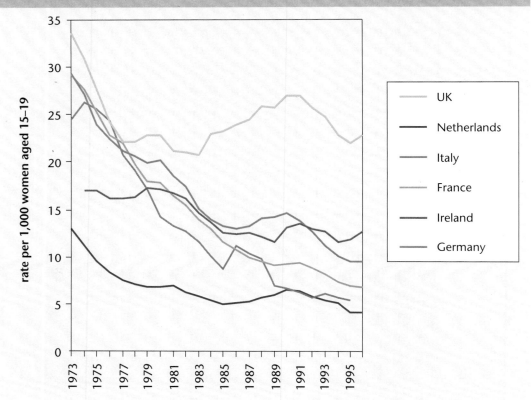

Source: Eurostat (Annex 1 refers).

Figure 4: Live birth rate to women aged 15–19: US, NZ, UK, Canada and Australia

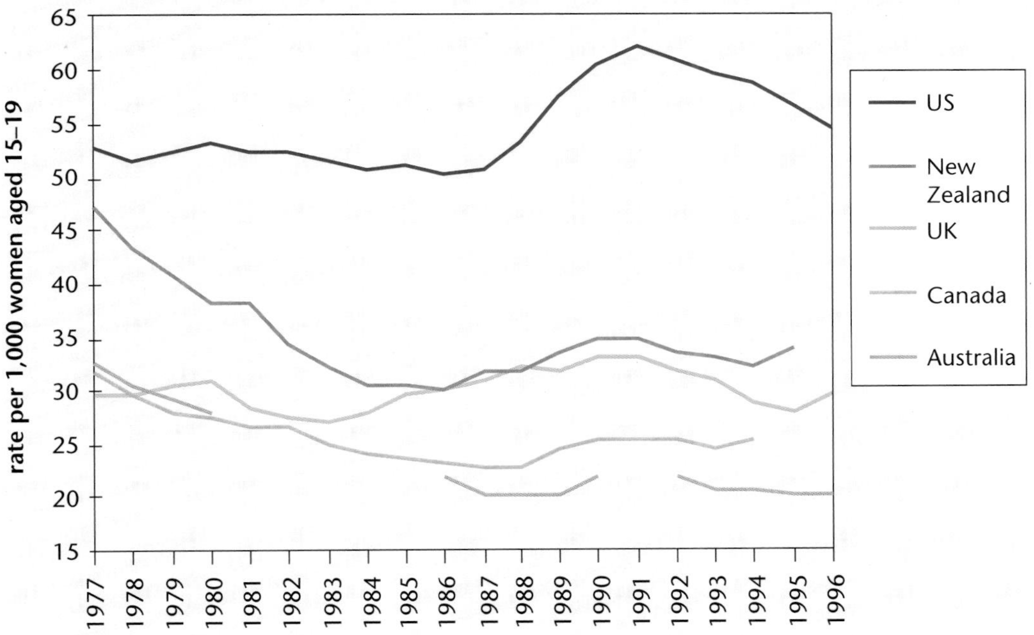

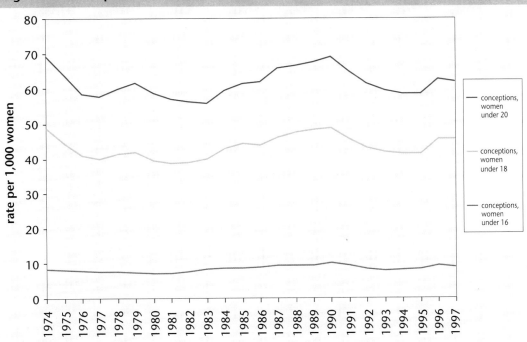

Source: Data collated by Centre for Sexual Health Research, University of Southampton (Annex 1 refers).

1.8 **Figure 5** shows the England picture in more detail. After a steep fall in the early and mid 1970s, the trend among under 20 year olds has been pretty much stuck at that level or higher. The conception rate among under 16s has been relatively stable during the whole period, but in 1997 the rate was 10 per cent higher than in 1993. Rates for all ages rose in 1996, probably as a result of the 1995 Pill scare.

Figure 5: Conception rates for women under 20, 18 & 16, England, 1974–1997

Source: ONS.

1.9 Over a third of all births are now outside marriage, but as **Figure 6** shows, for teenagers, the proportion is nearly 90 per cent. Twenty years ago it was around 40 per cent.

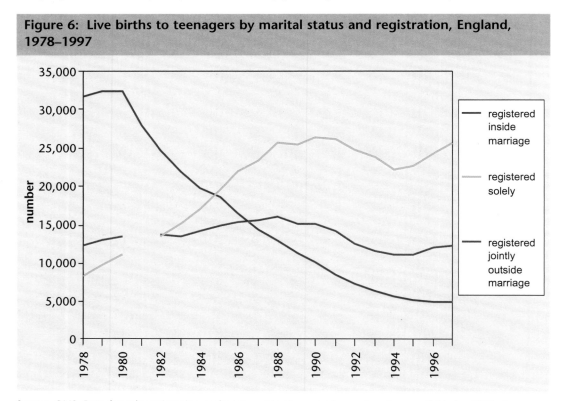

Figure 6: Live births to teenagers by marital status and registration, England, 1978–1997

Source: ONS. Data for sole registration and joint registration outside marriage is unavailable for 1981.

2. A SOCIAL EXCLUSION PHENOMENON?

> Teenage pregnancy is often a cause and a consequence of social exclusion. The risk of teenage parenthood is greatest for young people who have grown up in poverty and disadvantage or those with poor educational attainment. Overall, teenage parenthood is more common in areas of deprivation and poverty, but even the most prosperous areas have higher rates of teenage birth than the average in some comparable European countries.

Risk factors

2.1 Research in the United Kingdom and in other countries shows that young people with a history of disadvantage are at significantly greater risk of becoming parents in their teens.

- **Poverty** is a key risk factor. Research using the ONS Longitudinal Study has shown that the risk of becoming a teenage mother is almost *ten times* higher for a girl whose family is in social class V (unskilled manual), than those in social class I (professional).[7] Teenage girls who live in local authority or other social housing are three times more likely than their peers living in owner occupied housing to become a mother.[8]

- **Children in care** or leaving care have repeatedly been shown to be at higher risk of teenage pregnancy. Studies of the 1958 UK birth cohort found that women who had been in care or fostered were nearly two and a half times more likely than those brought up with both their natural parents to become teenage mothers.[9] For a more recent generation, one survey showed that a quarter of care leavers had a child by the age of 16,[10] and nearly half were mothers within 18 to 24 months after leaving care.[11]

- **Children of teenage mothers.** The daughter of a teenage mother is one and a half times more likely to become one herself than the daughter of an older mother.[12]

- **Educational problems.** Studies of both boys and girls in the 1958 UK birth cohort found that low educational achievement was a risk factor for teenage parenthood. Studies have found that girls with low attainment and those whose educational achievement *declined* between 7 and 16 were at greater risk than those whose achievement improved or was high at both ages.[13] In one recent small survey of nearly 150 teenage mothers in South London, more than 40 per cent left school with no qualifications – compared with a national average in England in 1997–98 of 6.6 per cent.[14] Girls who truant or are school excluded are also at relatively greater risk of becoming pregnant. One small study of 50 excluded girls showed that 14 per cent had become pregnant *during* their period of exclusion.[15]

- **Post 16.** There is evidence of a strong link between teenage parenthood and not being in education, training or work, for 16 and 17 year old women. In one study, almost half of non-participants were mothers, compared with 4 per cent who were in education, training or work. Further analysis suggested that about a third had become pregnant while not in education, training or work.[16]

- **Sexual abuse.** Several studies have shown an association between abuse in childhood and teenage pregnancy. US estimates suggest that the incidence of childhood physical or sexual abuse is about twice as high among pregnant teenagers as in the general population in the US.[17] Researchers put this down to a lack of confidence to resist sexual pressure – even years after the abuse. In this country, ChildLine report that about 5 per cent of the more than 7,000 calls they received about teenage pregnancy in 1996–97 also talked about sexual abuse.[18]

- **Mental health problems.** A number of recent studies have suggested a link between mental health problems and teenage pregnancy. In 1991, a study of 52 pregnant teenagers found that a quarter had a probable psychiatric disorder.[19] A 1991 follow-up study of 55 hospitalised adolescent girls with conduct disorders found that a third were pregnant before the age of 17.[20]

- **Crime.** There is also an association between involvement with the police and teenage parenthood. Studies of the 1958 UK birth cohort identified that teenage girls and boys who had been in trouble with the police had twice the risk of becoming a teenage parent than those who had no contact with the police.[21] It has been estimated that 25 per cent of the 11,000 prisoners in Young Offenders Institutions are fathers.[22] One Young Offenders Institution (Durham) estimates that around a third of its inmates are fathers.[23]

Multiple risk factors

2.2 Many young people share *several* of these risk factors and have a very high chance of becoming a teenage parent. One project for young parents run by Barnardos in Skelmersdale reported that of the young women in the project, 40 per cent had been in care, 70 per cent had lived with family breakdown, 40 per cent were the children of teenage mothers, but *all* had grown up in poverty, had done badly at school and had a history of not attending school.

2.3 The effect of multiple risk factors can be quantified in longitudinal surveys. Analysis of the 1958 UK birth cohort found that women with all the following characteristics had a 56 per cent chance of becoming a teenage mother, compared with a 3 per cent chance for those with none of them:[24]

A   emotional problems at 7 or 16;

B   mother was a teenage mother;

C   families who experienced financial adversity when they were 7 or 16;

D   a preference for being a young mother;

E   low educational attainment at 16.

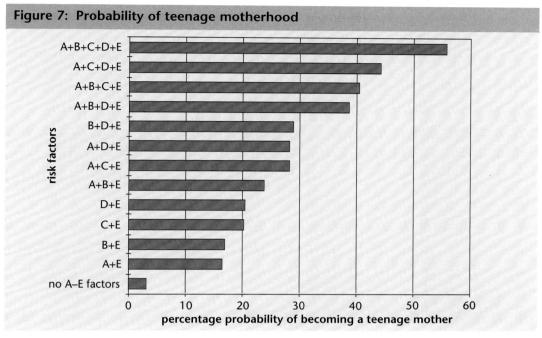

Figure 7: Probability of teenage motherhood

percentage probability of becoming a teenage mother

Source: K Kiernan, 1996.

Ethnic minorities

2.4 Multiple risk factors may also explain the over representation of some ethnic minorities amongst teenage parents, an issue which some ethnic minority groups highlighted in the Unit's consultation.

2.5 There are no comprehensive statistics on either live births or abortions by ethnic group because the mother's ethnic group is not recorded at birth registration or abortion. Information is collected on the mother's country of birth, but this does not identify women from ethnic minorities who were born in this country. However, we do have some information from the Labour Force Survey,[25] the Policy Studies Institute's report – The Fourth National Survey of Ethnic Minorities, 1994[26] and 'Health and Lifestyle Surveys',[27] conducted by the Health Education Authority (HEA). All of these surveys show that three ethnic minority groups in particular – Bangladeshis, African Caribbeans and Pakistanis – are at substantially greater risk of teenage parenthood than the national average.

2.6 The reasons for these variations are very complex, and further work on this should be a priority for future data gathering and research (see Annex 7 on the new research and information programme).

2.7 For some groups, the main driver may be traditions of early childbirth within marriage. A 1994 survey of Pakistani and Bangladeshi women in their 20s who had had a teenage birth found that over 90 per cent were or had been married, compared with 55 per cent for white women.[28] Surveys have reported that Pakistani and Bangladeshi women are least likely of all ethnic groups to have had sex before the age of 16.[29]

2.8 The link between disadvantage and early parenthood will also impact disproportionately on ethnic minority groups. For example, 41 per cent of African Caribbean, 82 per cent of Pakistani and 84 per cent of Bangladeshi people have incomes less than half the national average compared with 28 per cent of white people.[30] People from some ethnic minority groups are disproportionately likely to be in the acute risk groups listed above, for example in the care system or excluded from school. A number of groups consulted by the Unit said that sexual health services were frequently not designed in a way that would reach specific ethnic minority groups.

Area effects

2.9 Multiple risk factors also lead to a *geographical* concentration of teenage pregnancy. The poorest areas in England have teenage conception and birth rates up to six times higher than the most affluent areas.[31] **Figures 8 and 9** show how the teenage pregnancy map resembles the distribution of local authorities identified as the most deprived in the Unit's report on neighbourhood renewal.[32]

Figure 8: Under 18 conception rates by local authority district, England, 1997 (1998 boundaries)

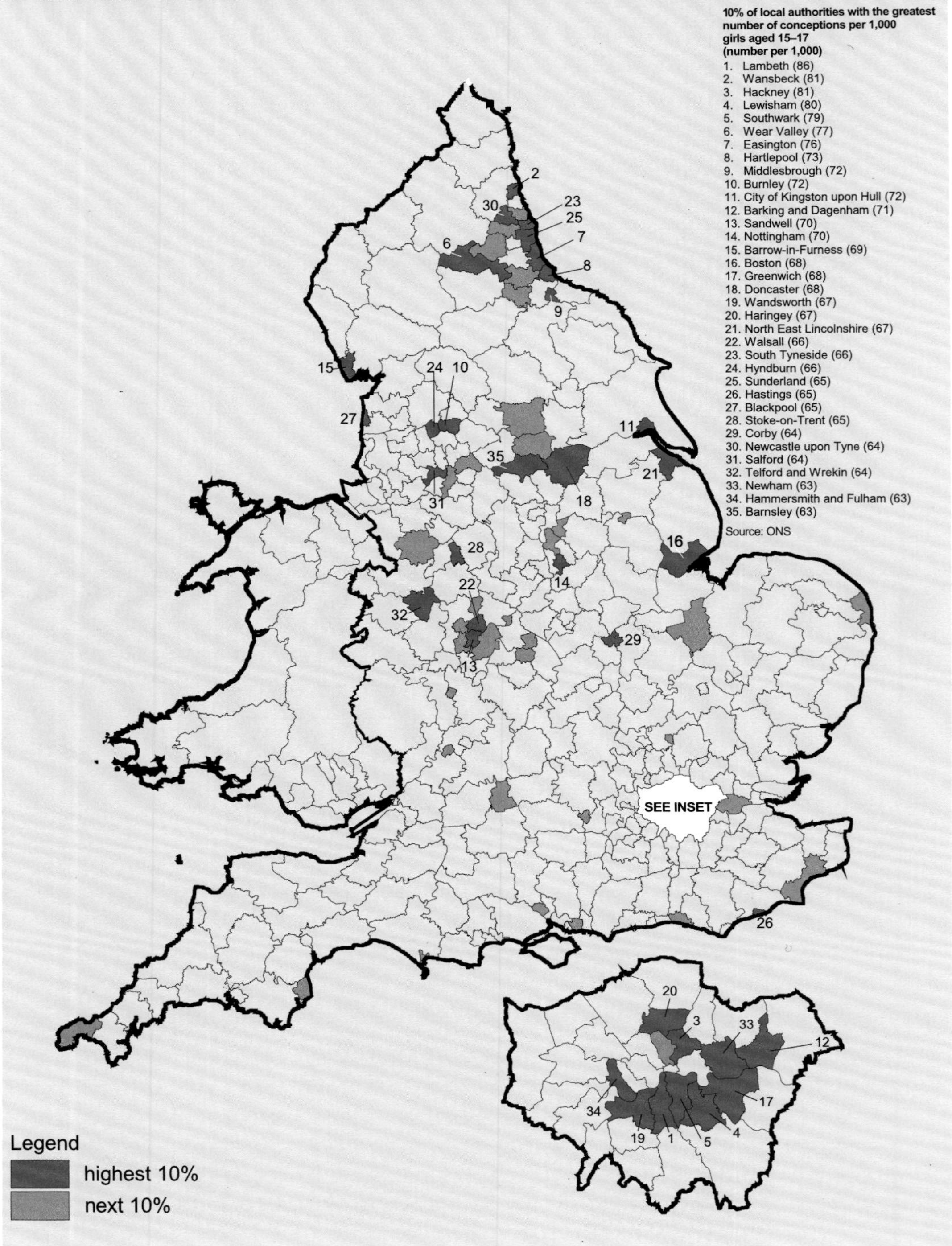

10% of local authorities with the greatest number of conceptions per 1,000 girls aged 15–17 (number per 1,000)

1. Lambeth (86)
2. Wansbeck (81)
3. Hackney (81)
4. Lewisham (80)
5. Southwark (79)
6. Wear Valley (77)
7. Easington (76)
8. Hartlepool (73)
9. Middlesbrough (72)
10. Burnley (72)
11. City of Kingston upon Hull (72)
12. Barking and Dagenham (71)
13. Sandwell (70)
14. Nottingham (70)
15. Barrow-in-Furness (69)
16. Boston (68)
17. Greenwich (68)
18. Doncaster (68)
19. Wandsworth (67)
20. Haringey (67)
21. North East Lincolnshire (67)
22. Walsall (66)
23. South Tyneside (66)
24. Hyndburn (66)
25. Sunderland (65)
26. Hastings (65)
27. Blackpool (65)
28. Stoke-on-Trent (65)
29. Corby (64)
30. Newcastle upon Tyne (64)
31. Salford (64)
32. Telford and Wrekin (64)
33. Newham (63)
34. Hammersmith and Fulham (63)
35. Barnsley (63)

Source: ONS

Legend

highest 10%

next 10%

Figure 9: Forty-four most deprived local authority districts in England according to the 1998 Index of Local Deprivation (in descending order of deprivation)

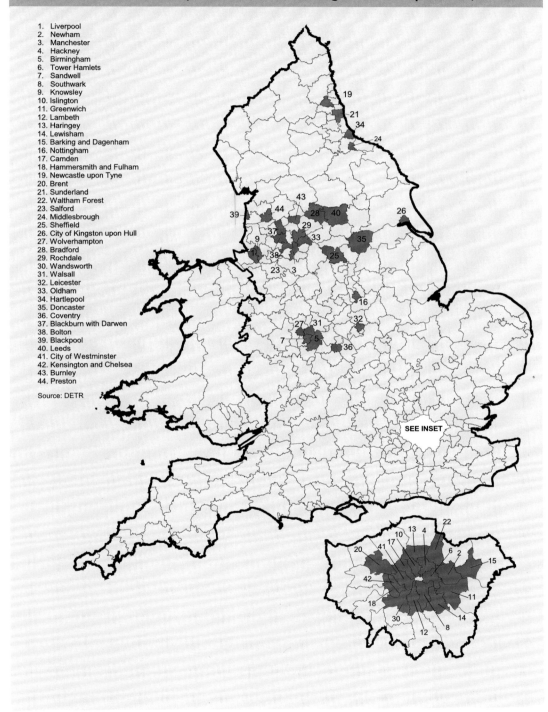

1. Liverpool
2. Newham
3. Manchester
4. Hackney
5. Birmingham
6. Tower Hamlets
7. Sandwell
8. Southwark
9. Knowsley
10. Islington
11. Greenwich
12. Lambeth
13. Haringey
14. Lewisham
15. Barking and Dagenham
16. Nottingham
17. Camden
18. Hammersmith and Fulham
19. Newcastle upon Tyne
20. Brent
21. Sunderland
22. Waltham Forest
23. Salford
24. Middlesbrough
25. Sheffield
26. City of Kingston upon Hull
27. Wolverhampton
28. Bradford
29. Rochdale
30. Wandsworth
31. Walsall
32. Leicester
33. Oldham
34. Hartlepool
35. Doncaster
36. Coventry
37. Blackburn with Darwen
38. Bolton
39. Blackpool
40. Leeds
41. City of Westminster
42. Kensington and Chelsea
43. Burnley
44. Preston

Source: DETR

2.10 But the match is not exact and deprivation is not the whole story. There are variations *between* seemingly equivalent areas, so Shropshire's teenage conception rate is more than 70 per cent higher than Cambridge and Huntingdon's[33] and **Figure 10** shows that even the most affluent areas usually have teenage birth rates that are higher than the national rates in, for example, the Netherlands or France.

Figure 10: Teenage birth rates for groups of English local authorities and national rates in Germany, France and the Netherlands, 1994

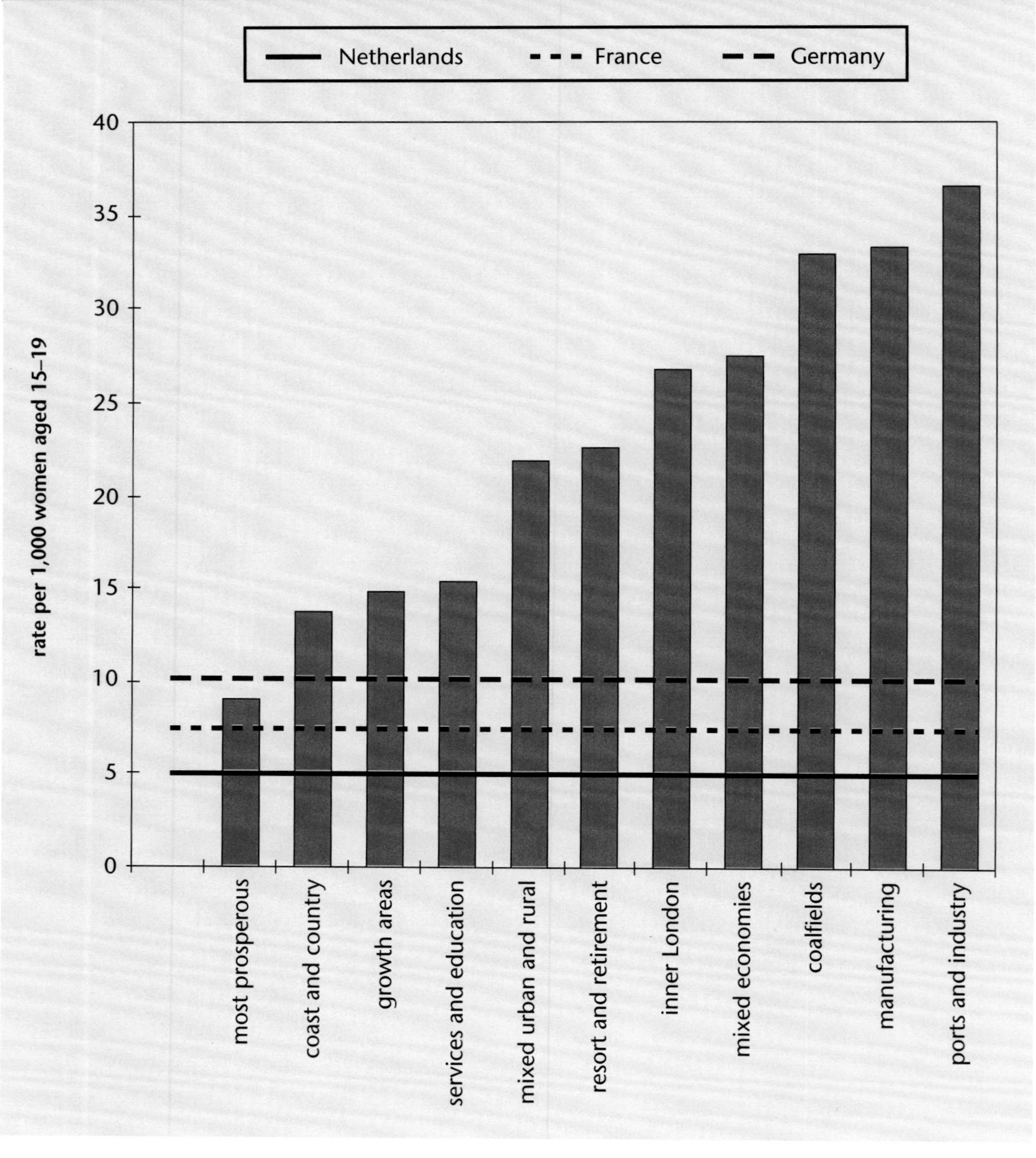

Sources: ONS and Eurostat.[34]

3. WHY DOES IT MATTER?

> **Teenage parents tend to have poor ante-natal health, lower birth weight babies and higher infant mortality rates. Their own health and their children's is worse than average. Teenage parents tend to remain poor and are disproportionately likely to suffer relationship breakdown. Their daughters are more likely to become teenage mothers themselves. Teenage mothers' usually disadvantaged backgrounds contribute to these effects. But having a baby young makes it worse.**

Health and welfare in pregnancy and after

3.1 Some obstetric risks are greater for young pregnant women, such as anaemia, toxaemia, eclampsia, hypertension, and prolonged and difficult labour.[35,36] There is also a greater chance of spontaneous abortions in subsequent pregnancies. On the other hand, these are arguably no more serious than many of the risks faced at the other end of the child bearing spectrum. Biologically, there is no reason why a teenage pregnancy should not have a good outcome if it is well managed.

3.2 The problem is that, because of their circumstances, teenage mothers tend not to have well managed pregnancies:

- ■ Teenagers usually go to their doctors much later in pregnancy (as three-quarters were not planning to become pregnant in the first place).[37]

- ■ For the same reason, they often miss out on important early pre-conception health measures such as taking folic acid supplements.[38]

- ■ During pregnancy, teenage mothers are the most likely of all age groups to smoke – see **Figure 11**. Nearly two-thirds of under 20s smoke before pregnancy and almost a half during it.[39]

- ■ For many, any kind of conventional ante-natal planning is an impossibility, as they face huge problems of family conflict, likely change of care or fostering arrangements, relationship stress or breakdown, and problems with education, housing and money.

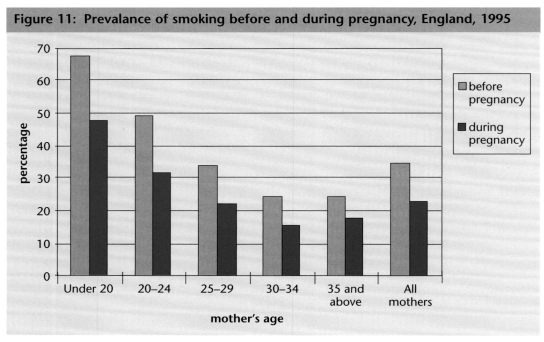

Figure 11: Prevalance of smoking before and during pregnancy, England, 1995

Legend: before pregnancy, during pregnancy

y-axis: percentage

x-axis: mother's age — Under 20, 20–24, 25–29, 30–34, 35 and above, All mothers

Source: ONS, Infant feeding survey 1995.

3.3 Many of these problems persist and intensify after the birth.

3.4 Relationship breakdown is more common among teenagers than those a few years older.[40] In one study, only around a half of teenage mothers were still in a relationship with the father a year after the baby's birth, with the other half usually without a steady partner.[41]

3.5 Teenagers are more likely to have to move house during pregnancy; one study showed that 17 per cent of teenage mothers moved three or more times during pregnancy or after the birth.[42] They often live in poor housing.[43] Nearly a third of teenage mothers are living alone with their baby a year after the birth.[44]

3.6 Teenage parents usually have low incomes. Ninety per cent receive Income Support; teenage parents are more likely than lone mothers generally to rely on benefits alone, and as **Figure 12** shows, teenage lone parents are likely to be stuck on benefits for longer spells than other lone parents.[45]

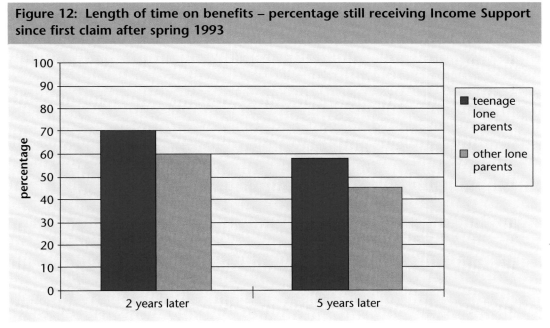

Figure 12: Length of time on benefits – percentage still receiving Income Support since first claim after spring 1993

Source: DSS analysis.

Outcomes

3.7 There are many individual success stories, where parents and children cope well and do well in the long run. But more often than not, the effects of long spells on benefit, poor education, no work, stress and relationship breakdown have a long term negative effect on teenage parents.

3.8 As a group, teenage mothers and their babies experience significant health deficits:

- ■ Teenage mothers are 25 per cent more likely than average to have a baby weighing less than 2,500 grams.[46]

- ■ The infant mortality rate for babies of teenage mothers in the first year of their lives is 60 per cent higher than for babies of older mothers.[47]

- ■ Mortality rates for both infants and children in the 1–3 age group are highest for mothers in the under 20 age group.[48]

- ■ Post-natal depression is three times as common amongst teenage parents, with four out of ten teenage mothers affected.[49]

- ■ Teenage mothers are only half as likely as older mothers to breastfeed.[50]

- ■ Children of teenage mothers are more likely to suffer accidents – especially poisoning or burns – and twice as likely to be admitted to hospital as the result of an accident or gastro-enteritis.[51]

3.9   Research on the 1958 UK birth cohort, examining the impact of childhood poverty and age at first birth on adult outcomes, found that early motherhood was strongly associated with adverse outcomes in later life (controlling for childhood poverty and a wide range of other background factors). Giving birth under 23 produced dramatic differences but giving birth as a teenager was usually associated with even higher risks of adverse outcomes.[52] This research and other studies found that those who became mothers in their teens:

- were more likely to have no qualifications by age 33;[53]

- were more likely to be in receipt of non-universal state benefits at age 33;[54]

- were likely to be on substantially lower incomes in their thirties than any other group, with nearly half in the bottom fifth of the income distribution;[55]

- if working, were more likely by mid twenties to be in semi-skilled or unskilled manual occupations;[56]

- were less likely to be home owners by the age of 33;[57]

- were more likely to have divorced or separated by the age of 33;[58] and

- were more likely to have large families by the age of 33 (20 per cent had four or more children by the age of 33).[59]

3.10 In turn, their children were:

- if daughters, more likely to become teenage mothers themselves;[60,61]

- more likely to have experience of a lone parent family[62] and the separation of their parents;[63,64] and

- at increased risk of living in poverty, living in poor housing and having bad nutrition.[65,66,67]

Poverty or age?

3.11 It has been argued that these poor outcomes are more the result of poverty rather than teenage parenthood. It is certainly true that whatever the age of the mother, poverty has an impact on a child's prospects. But as **Figure 13** shows, though infant mortality is higher for the poorest at all ages, a teenage birth worsens the risk for all social classes.

3.12 Childhood poverty was also associated with poor outcomes in adult life (net of age at first birth and other childhood factors) in research on the 1958 UK birth cohort, although generally not as strongly as the association of early motherhood with adverse outcomes. As **Figure 14** shows, age at first birth and poverty were mutually reinforcing. The worst outcomes were experienced by those who were poor *and* gave birth as a teenager.

Figure 13: Infant mortality by father's social class and mother's age, England and Wales, 1994–1996

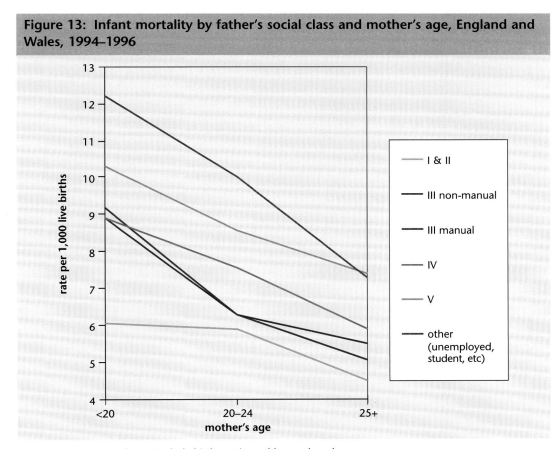

Source: ONS. Figures do not include births registered by mother alone.

Figure 14: Later life outcomes – effects of teenage birth and of clear childhood poverty

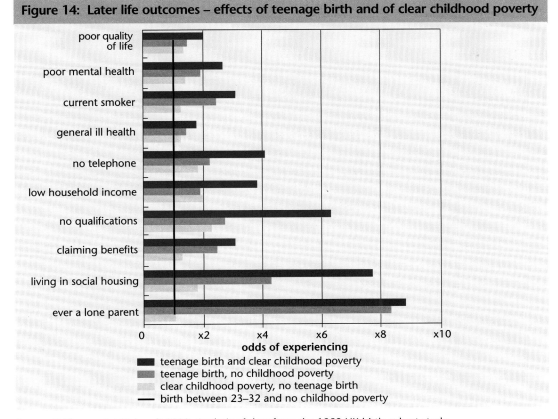

Source: K Kiernan & J Hobcraft 1999. Analysis of data from the 1958 UK birth cohort study.

4. WHY ARE RATES IN THE UK SO HIGH?

> The UK's relatively high rates of teenage pregnancy have many causes. Contraception use amongst teenagers is low by international standards. Social and economic factors also have a role to play. The UK and other countries with high rates of teenage pregnancy tend to be characterised by: high levels of income inequality; poor educational achievement; high percentages of lone parents; and benefit systems that do not require lone parents to be available for work until their children have left school.

"So people don't know about contraceptives?"

"They are aware but just can't be bothered."

"I think younger ones aren't aware that you can get it."

"They aren't aware of how easy it is to get pregnant and how hard it is to look after a baby."

"It depends what area they're living in again, because if it's somewhere like [...] they've not really got things to want to give it up. If you're in somewhere like [...] you'd probably want to go to University, so you wouldn't want a baby would you? But in [...] you've not really got anything like that."

"People were thinking, 'Oh, she only did it to get a council flat'. I had to wait ages for my flat. I cried when I saw it because it was so disgusting and dismal. It was utterly horrible. A complete tip. There was damp, mould, old furniture and broken glass."

"If I'd known what it was like, I would have waited another six years."

4.1 The UK's high rates of teenage pregnancy result from many factors, including ignorance, low expectations, mixed messages and a history of neglect.

Planned or unplanned

4.2 Most pregnant teenagers are pregnant because of accidents. Surveys find that around three-quarters of teenage mothers say their pregnancies are unplanned, and that the older teenagers are when they get pregnant, the more likely it is that the pregnancy was planned.[68,69,70] In practice, the first conscious decision that many teenagers make about their pregnancy is whether to have an abortion or to continue with the pregnancy.

Why so many accidents?

4.3 The average age of first sex in the UK is not markedly out of line with other European countries, which have lower rates of teenage pregnancy than the UK, or with the US, which has falling rates.

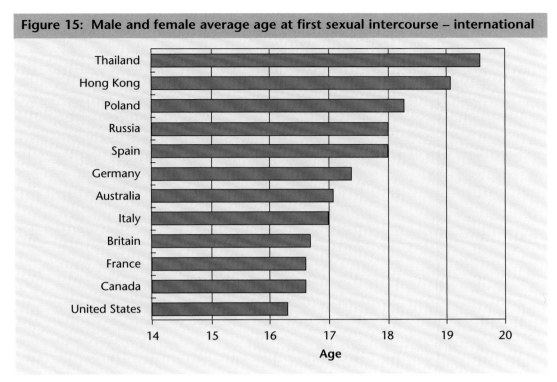

Figure 15: Male and female average age at first sexual intercourse – international

Source: Durex Global Sex Survey, 1998.

4.4 But the use of contraception by sexually active teenagers is low here compared with other European countries, as the table below shows.[71,72] The reasons young people give for this – ignorance about contraception, lack of access, lack of confidence in discussing it with a partner – are set out more fully in Chapter 7.

Table 1: Proportion of adolescents using contraception at first intercourse		
Netherlands	85 per cent	("young people")
Denmark	80 per cent	(15–16s)
Switzerland	80 per cent	("adolescents")
US	78 per cent	("adolescents")
France	74 per cent	(girls; 79 per cent boys (condom use))
New Zealand	75 per cent	(sexually active teenagers)
UK	50 per cent	(under 16s); 66 per cent (16–19s)

Abortions

4.5 Given the high level of accidental pregnancies, it is surprising that the UK does not have a higher number of abortions. **Figure 16** shows where the United Kingdom stands compared to other countries.[73]

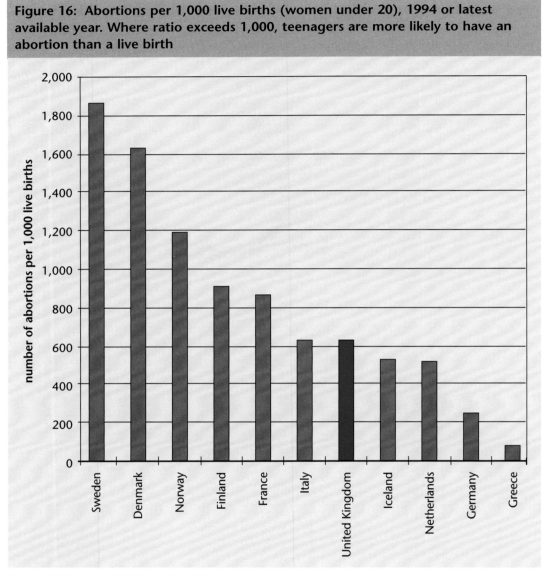

Figure 16: Abortions per 1,000 live births (women under 20), 1994 or latest available year. Where ratio exceeds 1,000, teenagers are more likely to have an abortion than a live birth

Source: UN Demographic Yearbooks 1996.

4.6 Chapter 8 shows that abortion numbers are heavily influenced by type of area; that in the poorest areas, young women tend to have fewer abortions, and are more likely to disapprove of abortion; and stigma attaching to abortion seems to outweigh apprehension about the idea of raising a child on their own and without a partner.

Social and economic factors

4.7 It has often been suggested that some pregnant teenagers decide to keep their baby so that they can claim benefit and housing. This is an unprovable assertion:

- Unsurprisingly researchers have never found any young women who said that benefits were their motivation, although some young people claimed to know of others who had.[74,75]

- A recent study of teenage parents found that most of the teenage mothers in their survey had only a hazy idea of what benefits they were entitled to when they were pregnant.[76]

4.8 A number of other factors make it seem **improbable:**

- As Chapter 9 sets out, the benefits available to a young parent are not generous, and most of the young people the Unit talked to were finding it extremely hard to manage.

- Relatively few young lone parents actually live in council flats – it is estimated that only 2,000 16–17 year old lone parents have sole tenancy,[77] mainly in social housing, though more are on the waiting list.

- Some of the areas with highest rates of teenage pregnancy now have council housing surpluses, admittedly of the least desirable property, and even without a baby, young people may be able to get a tenancy fairly readily.[78]

4.9 On the other hand, there is **some evidence** that:

- many young people find it much harder to cope as a teenage parent than they had expected (they may have expected the support available to be more generous than it is); and

- internationally, there is some association between countries with low levels of teenage parenthood and benefit systems that do require lone parents to be available for work before their children have reached their teens. Annex 6 provides more information on this area.[79]

4.10 Perhaps the best way to look at benefits and housing is as part of the context in which a pregnant young woman must make decisions about her future.

4.11 A teenager who:

- has a financially and emotionally secure background; and

- sees a clear future for herself through education or work;

has something to lose from early parenthood, and would probably see life on benefit very much as third or fourth best.

4.12 But the alternatives will look very different to a teenager who:

- ■ has grown up in poverty and possibly on benefits;

- ■ has had difficult family relationships, is in care, or is under pressure to move out; and

- ■ sees no prospect of a job and expects to be on benefit one way or the other.

For such a teenager, being a parent could well seem to be a better future than the alternatives.

International comparisons

4.13 The international evidence tells a similar story.

4.14 There is a striking correlation between countries with high rates of live births to teenagers and high levels of relative deprivation, dropping out of education, and family breakdown. The charts below show this clearly.

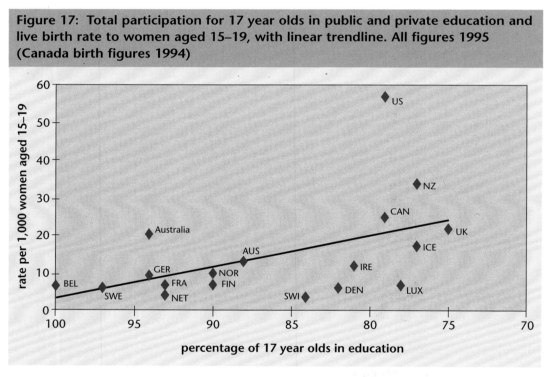

Figure 17: Total participation for 17 year olds in public and private education and live birth rate to women aged 15–19, with linear trendline. All figures 1995 (Canada birth figures 1994)

Source: Eurostat, Centre for Sexual Health Research, Southampton and OECD.

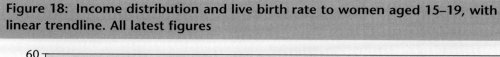

Figure 18: Income distribution and live birth rate to women aged 15–19, with linear trendline. All latest figures

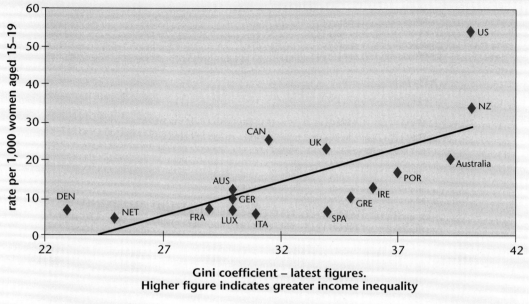

Source: Eurostat, Centre for Sexual Health Research, Southampton.

Figure 19: Lone parents as a percentage of all families and live birth rate to women aged 15–19, with linear trendline. All latest available figures

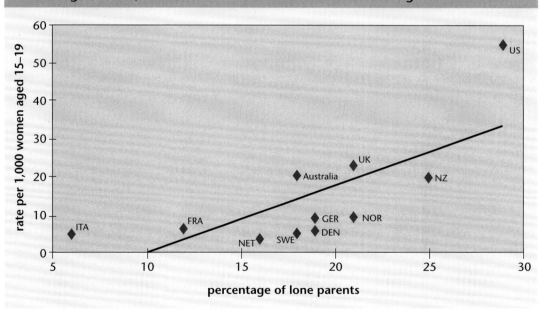

Source: Bradshaw et al 1996, Eurostat and Centre for Sexual Health Research, Southampton.

4.15 Countries which report low or falling rates of teenage parenthood tend to have a varied range of practical programmes to reduce the amount of under-age unprotected sex. These tend to focus on the provision of:

- adequate sex education and information;
- contraceptive services;
- postponement of sexual activity;
- 'life option' programmes to give alternatives to early parenting;
- assertiveness training and communication about contraception;
- problem solving and decision making skills; and
- improving family communication about sex.[80]

4.16 The effect of different factors is rarely easy to disentangle in any particular case. In the 1970s or 1980s, teenage birth rates in Sweden, the Netherlands, Switzerland, Denmark, Germany, Spain and Italy fell by a half or more. In these places, the falls coincided in part with greater access to contraception, bolstered by publicity campaigns encouraging its use and, more recently, AIDS campaigns that reinforced the messages to young people about the need to protect themselves from AIDS and other STIs.[81]

4.17 On the other hand, the 12 per cent drop in rates of 15–19 births in the US between 1991 and 1996 has been attributed to the health of the economy and better job prospects, fear of AIDS, the popularity of long lasting contraceptive methods such as implants and injectables, and more conservative attitudes to sex.[82]

4.18 Further information on international experience is set out in Annex 6. The chapters that follow set out in more detail, for this country, what is known about young people's experience of sex and pregnancy, starting with what they learn about sex and relationships and where they learn it from.

5. HOW MUCH DO TEENAGERS KNOW ABOUT SEX?

Research shows that ignorance about sex is a risk factor for teenage pregnancy and that good sex education helps to delay rather than accelerate when young people start sex. But parents are given little help to talk to their children about sex, and school-based sex education is patchy and often under-developed. Many teenagers lack information or rely on friends or the media. There is a considerable level of ignorance and misinformation among some teenagers about sex and its consequences, and how to deal with puberty and adolescence.

"Our lessons were taught by the head of RE. She seemed embarrassed talking about it."

"They just tell you about during the pregnancy, if they told you what it was going to be like after, not going out, trying to find a baby-sitter on a Saturday night. That would put a load of kids off anyway, not being able to go out drinking."

"The only sex education I had was an hour, somebody churning on about a condom. Nothing that helped me."

"They told us what the bits were called and my teacher was a nervous wreck."

"In school, we weren't taught anything... nothing was said about real feelings, or what happens if you get a girl pregnant."

"If someone came in and gave me a baby to look after for a day, I wouldn't have fell pregnant."

"They probably had something at my school, but I wasn't there for it. I was never there."

"My boyfriend really really wants to sleep with me, but he said he won't wear a condom, but if I drink vinegar...I won't get pregnant. Is this true?"

"I'm not used to the other sex, so I just can't talk to my son about sex."

"I ignored my own child's sexuality until I was confronted by her pregnancy. I don't want to make the same mistake with my other two younger children."

"As parents we suffer embarrassment because we have no role models to draw on, we ourselves were not taught about sex."

"I don't want my children to experience all the negative feelings that I experienced during puberty – feeling stupid, alone, confused."

How important is information about sex?

5.1 Research in this country and abroad shows that:

■ ignorance about sex is a key risk factor for teenage pregnancy (doubling the risk, according to one 1991 study);[83]

■ those who learn about sex mainly from school are less likely to become sexually active under age than those whose family and friends were their main source;[84]

■ good, comprehensive sex and relationships education (SRE) does not make young people more likely to start sex. Indeed it can help them delay starting sex, and make them more likely to use contraceptives when they do;[85,86,87,88,89]

■ the likelihood of teenage pregnancy is more than doubled for young women who did not discuss sex easily with their parents;[90]

■ over 90 per cent of parents and children look to schools as the favoured route for sex education;[91,92] and

■ in a 1991 survey of 19,000 people, two-thirds thought they should have been better informed about sex when they started being sexually active; of these, a third of the women and half of the men wanted more sex education from school.[93]

How good is information about sex?

5.2 The Unit heard of much good practice in SRE during its consultations. But overall it found that:

■ in some schools, SRE is an under resourced subject, squeezed for time, not supported by training, and not attached to wider local strategies to combat teenage pregnancy or improve sexual health;

■ parents are given very little help in talking to their children about sex at home; and

■ although there are some good examples of projects to reach teenagers in youth and community settings, they are unevenly spread throughout the country and are poorly funded.

5.3 This has two consequences. First, *young people pick up information about sex where they can.* A 1997 survey found that, for children of 14 and 15, friends were as influential a source of information about sex as was school.[94] And on sexual health issues such as STIs, a 1998 survey showed that, among young people and teenagers:

■ no less than 68 per cent learned about them from the media (including advertising);

■ 13 per cent learned from friends or relatives; and

■ only 18 per cent learned the facts from doctors, clinics or other sources.[95]

5.4 There has been a rapid increase in children's unsupervised access to media such as TV and the Internet. It is estimated that two-thirds of all children have televisions in their bedrooms.[96]

5.5 Second, *young people are frequently ignorant or misinformed* about sex and their own physical development:

- In one survey, a third of girls said they had not been told by their parents about periods before they started (and one in ten had not been told by anyone).[97]

- Of nearly 4,000 14 and 15 year olds surveyed recently by the Health Education Authority (HEA), over a quarter thought the Pill protected against STIs, and a similar proportion thought the same about having a steady partner.[98]

5.6 These weaknesses affect more than the minority who have sex and get pregnant in their teens, and teenagers know this: the universal message the Unit received from young people during its consultation is that the sex and relationships education they receive falls far short of what they would like to equip them for managing relationships as they grow into adulthood. Certainly the huge number of calls to helplines like Sexwise (see Chapter 10), and the enduring popularity of problem pages in teen magazines points to a great unmet need among teenagers for basic, factual information about sex.

Sources of sex education: schools

The law

5.7 The legal framework for sex education is very complex. The basic biology – puberty, where babies come from and so on – is part of the science national curriculum. The broad requirements are set out in the box overleaf. Particularly at key stage 2 (the last years of primary school) they are open to a broad range of interpretations.

5.8 More broadly, sex education is seen as falling under the legal requirements for schools to provide a curriculum which:

- promotes the spiritual, moral, cultural, mental and physical development of pupils at the school and of society; and

- prepares such pupils for the opportunities, responsibilities and experiences of adult life.

5.9 **Primary schools** in England are required by law to have a policy on sex education (though this does not mean that they have to *teach it*: the policy could be *not to do so*). Around 10 per cent of primary schools do not have a policy,[99] although the Department for Education and Employment (DfEE) is encouraging all schools to do so.

SEX EDUCATION IN THE NATIONAL CURRICULUM

Within the National Curriculum for science, pupils should be taught:

at key stage 1 (5–7)
- that humans move, feed, grow, use their senses and reproduce;

- to name the main external parts of the human body;

- that humans grow from babies into children and then into adults, and that adults can produce babies; and

- to recognise similarities and differences between themselves and other pupils.

at key stage 2 (7–11)
- that there are life processes common to all animals; and

- the main stages of the human life cycle, growth and reproduction.

at key stage 3 (11–14)
- that living things have structures that enable life processes to take place;

- the ways in which some cell types, including sperm and ovum are adapted to their functions;

- the human reproductive system, menstrual cycle, fertilisation, and the role of the placenta;

- how the foetus develops in the uterus;

- the physical and emotional changes that take place during adolescence; and

- that bacteria and viruses can affect health.

at key stage 4 (14–16)
- that the nucleus contains chromosomes that carry the genes;

- the way in which hormonal control occurs, including the effects of insulin and sex hormones;

- the medical use of hormones, including the control and promotion of fertility and the treatment of diabetes;

- how variation may arise from both genetic and environmental causes;

- that sexual reproduction is a source of genetic variation while asexual reproduction produces clones;

- how gender is determined in humans; and

- the basic principles of genetic engineering, cloning and selective breeding.

5.10 Maintained **secondary schools** are required by law to *make provision* for sex education for all registered pupils. Sex education is not fully defined in the law, but it must include education about HIV/AIDS and other STIs. Parents have a legal *right to withdraw* their children from sex education, except those parts that are within the National Curriculum (the National Curriculum covers teaching about hormonal forms of contraception which affect the body, such as the Pill or injections). Around 1 per cent of parents use the right to withdraw their children. Many of those parents see this right as an important way of ensuring that their children are brought up in accordance with their faith or culture. Removal of the right would require a change to legislation, which is not currently being considered.

Guidance

5.11 The DfEE issued guidance in 1994 on the content and purpose of sex education.[100] This guidance made a number of points about process and factors that schools should bear in mind in designing policies. But it had little to say about what materials or information were appropriate at what stage. This advice gives considerable latitude to schools on the scope, quality and time spent on SRE, and this fact is reflected in the comments received by the Unit from young people, teachers and parents.

Practice

5.12 In most schools SRE forms part of wider provision often grouped under the title Personal, Social and Health Education. This is not part of the National Curriculum. It is a developing discipline for which no specialist qualification exists.

5.13 In **primary schools**, practice seems to vary widely. Some schools do nothing, with the result that girls start their periods with no idea what is happening to them and a small minority become sexually active before they have received any sex education at all. On the other hand, some primary schools provide detailed and extensive programmes from quite early ages.

5.14 Most of the teachers who teach SRE or the wider PSHE are primarily teachers of another curriculum subject, although the school nurse or other health professionals can play a valuable role in promoting and teaching SRE; their clinical training and pastoral activity giving them added credibility with pupils when discussing sex and contraception. With the consent of the governors, some school nurses also provide confidential advice to pupils on a range of issues, including sex, and can act as a bridge to GP and other medical services for young people including, where appropriate, emergency contraception.

5.15 SRE is not automatically included in OFSTED inspections. Inspectors may inspect lessons if they are being taught while other inspections are taking place, but this is not mandatory.

What pupils think

5.16 Generally, young people tell researchers they feel they are told too little, too late. A recent survey of school pupils showed that they believed that learning to say "no" was the most important, and the first thing they should learn in SRE.[101] Teenagers themselves repeatedly told the Unit and other researchers that sex education is unsuccessful with their age group because it addresses only the mechanics of sex, rather than self confidence and esteem and how to talk about feelings.[102,103] Boys in particular have said that the way sex education is taught makes it hard for them not to giggle and laugh in embarrassment. They did not feel able to ask questions about relationships or sex.

What schools think

5.17 Many of those involved in SRE are concerned that those who innovated would become the subject of unwelcome media attention. Several school heads said that although they were proud of the quality of their school's SRE, they did not want, for this reason and because of the possible reaction from parents, to become known as 'good schools' for sex education.

Parents

5.18 Parents tell researchers that the more they know about a school's sex education programme, the more satisfied they are with it, but over a third in one study said that they had never been consulted on the delivery of sex education to their children.[104]

5.19 **Figure 20** shows that compared with the Netherlands, families in this country seem reluctant to talk to their children about sex and relationships.[105] During the Unit's consultation, parents repeatedly said that they felt embarrassed and ill-equipped to broach this subject with their children, and this was made worse for many by knowing little about what was taught at school.

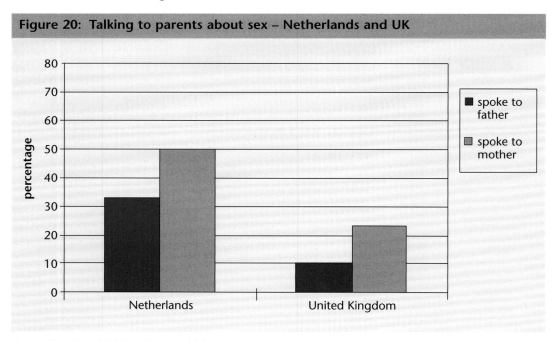

Figure 20: Talking to parents about sex – Netherlands and UK

Source: R Ingham & G Van Zessen, 1998.

5.20 Although there are some individual projects that provide support and advice to parents on how to address issues of sex and sexual health, most receive nothing.

5.21 The picture that emerges in the following chapters – of growing numbers of quite young teenagers drifting into sexual relationships with haphazard use of contraception – highlights weaknesses in the sex and relationships education that young people in this country receive, whether from school or home.

5.22 The boxes in Chapter 10 detail projects visited by the Unit which show promise in tackling the problems set out in this chapter.

6. TEENAGERS' EXPERIENCE OF SEX

> The pressures on teenagers to have sex are growing and the age at which they become sexually active has decreased. They are pressured to have sex by their peers, and by a belief that it is expected of them. Sex among teenagers is often opportunistic, unplanned, affected by alcohol and takes place outside of any long term commitment. A tiny group begin to have sex before they are even in their teens.

"It's a race isn't it?"

"At school trying not to be last in class to lose it."

"It is. That's what we were like at school. I were 14 when I lost my virginity and when I think back I didn't use any protection, was not on the Pill or anything. I was a bloody stupid idiot [...] I just wanted to race with everyone else."

"I didn't feel ready, all my friends egged me on by telling me that it was excellent and that they had all done it. Half of them haven't; they wanted me to do it so I could tell them all about it."

"They persuade you don't they?"

"If you really like him you're going to do it aren't you?"

"Otherwise they're going to split up with you. And you don't want them to because you really like them or something like that."

"You need to display a macho image to impress the lasses: 'you must be gay if you're not sleeping with your girlfriend.'"

"It was really good.... went round the school pretty quick. It was one up on the notch, wasn't it?"

"I was scared before anything, but when I first met her I was a bit drunk and she was a bit drunk and we'd just gone back from a party to her place and it just happened."

"I thought that once you were going out with a bloke you had to sleep with them, that was the process. I really thought that. And you didn't. And I was thinking that I have to make the move before they do."

"You think everybody is doing that and they ain't. It's only afterwards you think 'what do you mean you haven't? I wish I hadn't. I thought you had.'"

"I should have, like, saved it. I would like to be able to say that I was 16 and that it was nice."

"I just wanted to get it over and done with so I could say 'yeah, I've done it' and now I can find a bloke who likes me and maybe it will be better."

6.1 The average age at which young people start having sex has been getting younger. It is now 17; forty years ago it was 21 for women and 20 for men.[106]

6.2 **Figure 21** shows how the numbers of young people sexually active by age 16 doubled between 1965 and 1991, with the rise most striking for girls. Some more recent estimates put the numbers sexually active before age 16 as high as one in three.[107]

6.3 The HEA estimate that among sexually active 16–19 year olds, just over a quarter of boys and nearly a half of girls had had two or more sexual partners in the last year.[108]

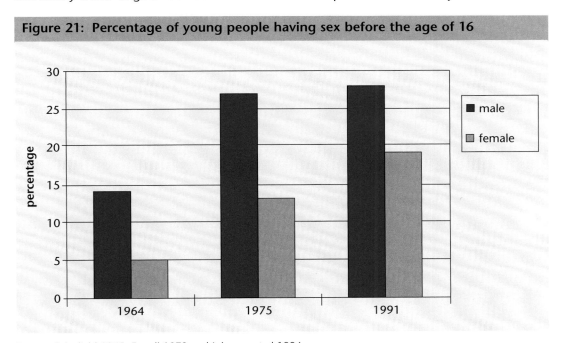

Figure 21: Percentage of young people having sex before the age of 16

Source: Schofield 1965, Farrell 1978 and Johnson et al 1994.

6.4 Some of the fall in age of first intercourse may reflect falling ages of sexual maturity, thanks to improvements in general health and diet. There is no consensus on exactly what the average age of puberty now is for young women but teachers consistently report more girls starting their periods in primary schools,[109] and one study estimates the figure to be 10 per cent.[110] Girls themselves report a wide range of ages for starting periods – from 8 to 15, with an average of 12 years and 7 months.[111]

6.5 There is a very small group of young people who start having sex in their pre-teens; around 1 per cent of 11 and 12 year olds are sexually active.[112] The table below shows the number of abortions and births for girls under 14 over the last three years.[113] Some of these will be the result of sexual abuse.

Table 2: Abortions and live births by age, England 1995–1997		
Girl's age	Abortions 1995–97	Live births 1995–97
9	1	–
10	1	–
11	1	2
12	36	6
13	442	89

6.6 As **Figure 22** shows, those who begin sex before 16 are more than three times as likely to have a child before they are 20.

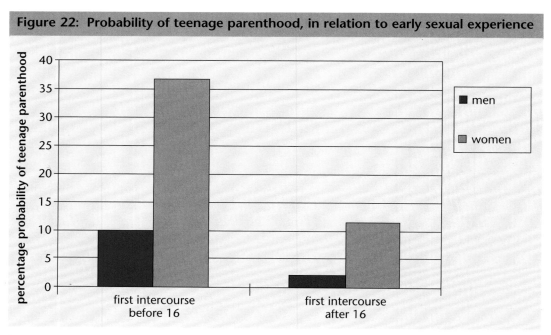

Figure 22: Probability of teenage parenthood, in relation to early sexual experience

Source: K Wellings et al, 1996. Data from the National Survey of Sexual Attitudes and Lifestyles.

First intercourse

6.7 As the quotations at the start of this chapter show, young people, parents and those working with young people give a variety of reasons for starting sex, including:

- curiosity;

- opportunity;

- real or imagined peer pressure;

- the wish not to be left behind;

- being in a relationship;

- fear of losing boy or girlfriend;

- the need to feel loved and the belief that sex equals love;

- media influences that glamorise sex; and

- alcohol.[114],[115]

6.8 The importance of alcohol in teenage sex is borne out by wider survey evidence, for instance a recent HEA study of 16–24 year olds showed that after drinking alcohol 1 in 5 have had sex that they later regretted, 1 in 7 have had unsafe sex, and 1 in 10 have been unable to remember whether they had sex the night before.[116]

Peer pressure

6.9 For some especially vulnerable young people, there will be a combination of many different factors at work, which leaves them at greater risk of pregnancy than others of their age. Both young men and women in care, for example, often feel pressurised by peers and partners to have sex. That extra pressure and enhanced opportunities (particularly in children's homes) can lead to starting sexual relationships at a relatively early age.

6.10 However, peer pressure to have sex is obviously a general problem amongst young people. The Unit's discussions with young people revealed significant uncertainty about what to expect in relationships, with young people of both sexes fitting in as much with what they thought others wanted as making their own choices and many reported great disappointment and regret after the event. In one survey, 6 out of 10 women believed, in retrospect, that having sex before 16 had been "too soon".[117]

Forced sex

6.11 There is some evidence from research abroad that a significant proportion of first sex is unwanted – that no positive choice is made to have sex, and that the younger the person is when they start having sex, the more likely it is that sex is unwanted. Surveys in the US put the proportion of first sex that is unwanted as high as 70 per cent for under 13s. A study of the 1972 birth cohort in New Zealand revealed that 7 per cent of women reported their first sex as forced; not just unwanted but forced upon them.[118]

International comparisons

6.12 **Figure 23** illustrates the results of a recent study which looked at the differences between teenage attitudes to sex in the Netherlands and the UK. The study analysed the results from 200 in-depth interviews with young people in both countries. Each interview covered a variety of topics, including the factors leading to first intercourse. These reasons were then sifted into the four broad categories shown. Many young people gave more than one factor. It shows that in the UK, for girls and even more so for boys, peer pressure and opportunity were much more likely to be factors in first intercourse and love and commitment much less so than for young people in the Netherlands.[119]

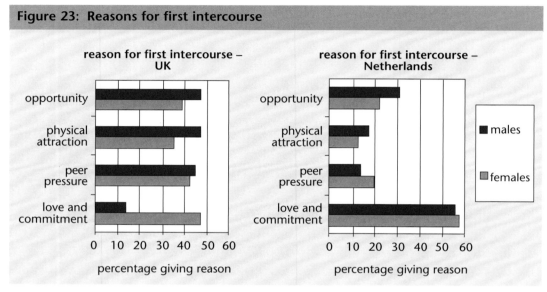

Figure 23: Reasons for first intercourse

Source: R Ingham, 1998.

Under-age sex and the law

6.13 The law makes it illegal for a man to have sexual intercourse with a girl under the age of 16 and the maximum penalty is two years imprisonment. For sexual intercourse with a girl under 13 years old, it is life imprisonment. But the number of reports of offences to the police has declined over the last 10 years, and police cautions and prosecutions by the Crown Prosecution Service (CPS) resulting in convictions have fallen in proportion, as **Figure 24** shows.

Figure 24: Unlawful sexual intercourse offences – girls under 13 and 16, England 1987 and 1997. Offences involving girls under 13 shown as a shaded proportion

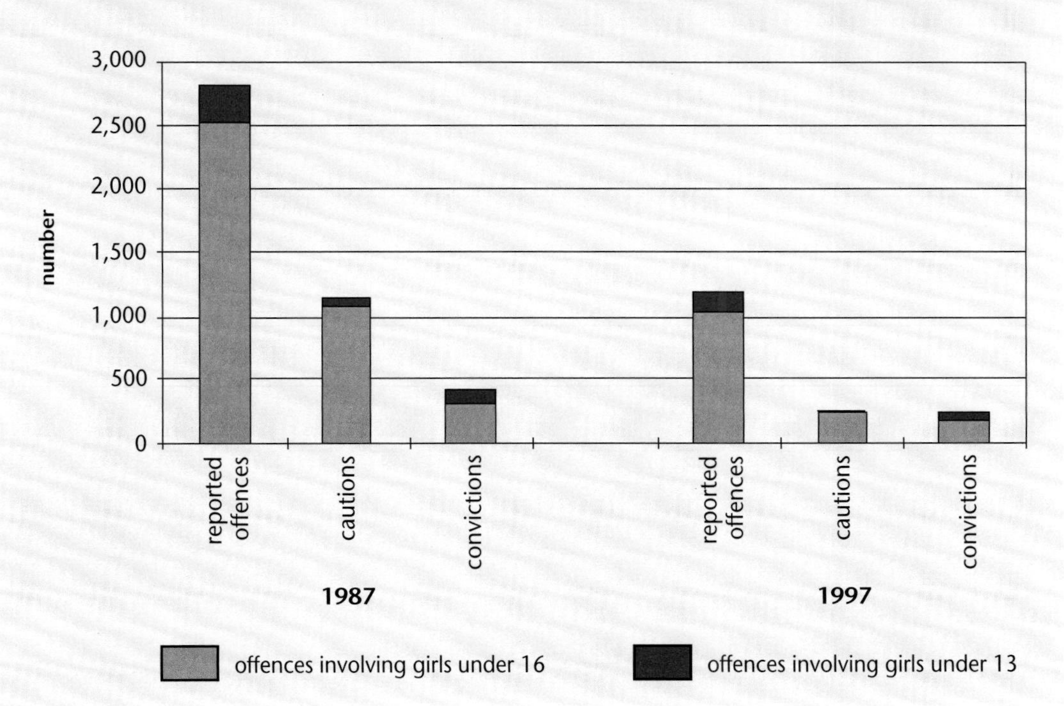

Source: Home Office. Cautions and convictions relate to offenders, not individual offences.

6.14 There is no defence to the offence of having sexual intercourse with a girl under 13, but Section 6 of the Sexual Offences Act 1956 allows two defences to the offence of sexual intercourse with a girl under the age of 16:

a   that the man reasonably believes the girl to be his wife; or

b   that the man is under 24, has not been charged with a like offence, and reasonably believes the girl to be over 16.

6.15 In deciding whether to prosecute, the CPS has to consider if there is a realistic prospect of conviction and if it is in the public interest to take the case to Court. The defence at b above makes it more difficult to show a realistic prospect of conviction when the man is under 24. The Code for Crown Prosecutors sets out factors to be taken into account when considering whether or not prosecution is in the public interest. Factors in favour of prosecution include where the defendant is in a position of trust or authority, and where the victim was vulnerable. So the wider the age gap, the more likely it is that prosecution should be found to be in the public interest.

6.16 The law on sex seems to have little effect on influencing young peoples' behaviour, and was hardly ever mentioned by young people during the Unit's consultation as a factor in a decision to begin sexual activity. As one put it:

> "If someone wants to have sex, they won't go 'ah, but I can't because I'll be breaking the law'. They'll just do it. [...] Alcohol, smoking, anything to do with the legal age is a load of crap. Nobody pays attention to it."

47

6.17 But a number of other people and organisations in the Unit's consultation expressed concern that while the law may not have an effect on teenagers' behaviour with each other, it might influence an older man's behaviour towards under-age girls if they know there is a ready, and broadly defined, defence they can deploy if charged with an offence. They have argued that possible cases of abuse involving a man up to 10 years older than an under-age girl risk not being investigated because of the present defence for men under 24. The child charity, Barnardos, through its work with children involved in, or at risk of, child prostitution, believes that the 10 year age range potentially encompassed within the 1956 Act is too great and will very likely involve a potential abuse of the girl – it believes an age range of five years would be more realistic.

6.18 The boxes in Chapter 10 detail projects visited by the Unit which show promise in tackling the problems set out in this chapter.

7. TEENAGERS AND CONTRACEPTION

> Between a third and a half of sexually active teenagers do not use contraception at first intercourse; a higher proportion than in many other European countries. A sexually active teenager who does not use contraception has a 90 per cent chance of conceiving over a year and teenage rates of STIs are rising fast. There is often greater embarrassment about using or discussing contraception than about sex itself. Teenagers are confused about *where* they can get contraceptive advice or treatment, *whether* it is legal for them to do so, and *how* to use it.

7.1   Sexually active teenagers not using contraception are taking severe risks:

   ■   They have a 90 per cent chance of conceiving in one year.[120]

   ■   In a single act of unprotected sex with an infected partner, teenage women have a 1 per cent chance of acquiring HIV, a 30 per cent risk of getting genital herpes and a 50 per cent chance of contracting gonorrhoea.[121]

   ■   Sixteen to nineteen year olds have the highest rate of increase in gonorrhoea of any age group, with a 45 per cent increase in new cases in 1995–1997 alone.[122]

   ■   One STI, chlamydia, affects teenage girls more than any other age group.[123] It is the biggest cause of ectopic pregnancy, and can lead to infertility. It can cause discharge and pain, but there are usually no symptoms, so the sufferer may never know they are infected. Diagnoses of chlamydia in Genito-Urinary Medicine clinics for 16–19 year olds rose by around 53 per cent between 1995 and 1997.[124]

   ■   The prevalence of genital warts amongst teenagers has also increased by a quarter over the same period.[125]

7.2   Despite these risks half of under 16s and a third of 16–19s in the UK use no contraception the first time they have sex[126] and many carry on not using it. The proportions not using contraception at first intercourse are up to double the rates in other countries as the table in Chapter 4 illustrated.

7.3   Teenagers who admit that they do not use contraception give a variety of reasons. In a study in 1994 of Scottish teenagers presenting for abortion, they gave the following reasons for not having used contraceptives:[127]

Table 3: Reasons for not having used contraceptives, Scottish study, 1994	
dislike/afraid of it	39 per cent
didn't think it would happen to me	21 per cent
unplanned intercourse	21 per cent
afraid parents would find out	19 per cent
afraid to ask doctor	19 per cent
don't understand them	16 per cent
father did not want or not discussed	16 per cent
other	17 per cent

7.4   What young people told the Unit during its consultations expands on these factors a little, and shows a complex picture where ignorance and reluctance to use contraceptives are combined with embarrassment about accessing them and problems with particular methods.

> *"You just think – well, nothing's going to happen to me, it's just a one-off thing, so you take the chance..."*

> *"I have used a condom, but I don't like it, it puts you off. What's the use of having sex if you don't enjoy it?"*

> *"My friend said her boyfriend was allergic to condoms. Now she's pregnant by him. She's 13."*

> *"When you don't use them, you're just so pissed out of your brains you don't know what you're doing so you just forget about it."*

> *"It's not until one of your friends catches a disease that you really take notice."*

> *"Clinics are so badly publicised. I walked past mine loads of times because it's just a little shop with blinds in the window."*

> *"I'd go to my GP."*
> *"I wouldn't. I couldn't do that. I know the nurses."*

> *"My mum did take me to the doctor. He refused to put me on the Pill. I was 13 years old, it was four weeks to my 14th birthday. I went back when I was 14, but I was already pregnant."*

> *"They just get you in and get you out again."*

"They've had that many, so many a day that they don't have time to talk to you."

"I'd forget to take them [the pills]. I'd miss a day."
"I missed days all the time."
"I just think of people dying of them and that."

"That's the most embarrassing thing that happened to my brother, he didn't know how to put a condom on when he first slept with his girlfriend."

"The clinic isn't open until Thursday night. I needed the morning-after pill one Sunday and ended up in the casualty department of the hospital. I had to go into the children's ward because I was under 16, so I was thinking, 'oh God, I'm going to be pregnant', looking at pictures of Teletubbies and Barney all over the walls."

7.5 Five particular issues about contraception that emerged from the Unit's consultation are worth highlighting:

(i)   Under 16s' confusion about the law

7.6 The law on under-age contraception is quite clear that under 16s:

■   have a right to confidentiality for their discussions with medical practitioners. Child protection procedures cover what to do in cases where there is an issue of abuse or exploitation;

■   should not fear being reported to their parents just for consulting a doctor; and

■   can obtain contraceptive treatment without parental consent if certain conditions are met (see box overleaf for more details).

7.7 Nonetheless, many sexually active teenagers have told researchers that they think their parents will be told if they try to obtain contraception, or that it is illegal to ask for contraception because it is illegal to have sex under age. In one survey in 1993, 66 per cent of pregnant teenagers said that they thought it illegal to go to either a GP or a family planning clinic.[128]

THE LAW ON MEDICAL TREATMENT FOR UNDER 16S

Under English law, the capacity of those under 16 to consent to their own treatment is governed by the common law. The leading case remains Gillick v West Norfolk and Wisbech Area Health Authority [1985] 3 AER 402. In that case, the House of Lords held that the law did not recognise any rule of absolute parental authority until a fixed age, and such rights yielded to children's rights to make their own decisions when they reached a sufficient understanding and intelligence to be capable of making up their own minds.

The Lords held that it followed that a doctor had discretion to give contraceptive advice or treatment to a girl under 16 without her parents' knowledge or consent, provided the girl had reached an age where she had sufficient understanding and intelligence to enable her to understand fully what was proposed. They also said that whether she did understand or not was a question of fact in each case.

This test for the capacity of the under 16s has come to be known informally as 'Gillick competence' and is applicable in a wide range of situations, not just in relation to medical treatment.

In England and Wales, section 8 of the Family Law Reform Act 1969 provides that those aged 16 and 17 may consent to their own medical, surgical or dental treatment and no consent need be given by a parent or other person with parental responsibility for that treatment.

Further guidance (Contraceptive Advice and Treatment for Young People Under 16, HC(86)1) was issued by the Department of Health after the Lords' judgment, which indicated that a doctor or other health professional providing contraceptive advice or treatment to an under 16 without parental consent should be satisfied that:

- the young person will understand the advice and the moral, social and emotional implications;

- the young person cannot be persuaded to tell their parents or allow the doctor to tell them that they are seeking contraceptive advice;

- the young person is having, or is likely to have, unprotected sex whether they receive the advice or not;

- their physical or mental health is likely to suffer unless they receive the advice or treatment; and

- it is in the young person's best interests to give contraceptive advice or treatment without parental consent.

(ii) Clinics and doctors

7.8 In 1996–97, 76,700 girls under 16 attended family planning clinics, while 31,000 were registered with a GP for family planning services (there may be some double counting in these figures).[129] Even where teenagers are aware of their rights under the law, a range of practical factors can then inhibit them from using the services that are available:

- *Location and opening hours* are critical for teenagers who may be tied to a school timetable and rely on public transport. One researcher has suggested that teenagers are more likely to use contraception if they are within a 30 minute bus ride, or 20 minute walk of a clinic.[130] For others, it is important to be able to use services that are further from home and where there is no chance of being recognised.

- The Unit was often told in its consultation that young people are intimidated by the *atmosphere* of many places that provide contraceptives. Young people have told of not being allowed to make an appointment with a GP without a parent present; of feeling that staff disapproved and made that clear; and of being given a 'ration' of condoms that was smaller than they needed. Better advertising, accessibility and improved privacy were seen by some as advantages of family planning clinics[131] compared with GPs, but others believed that family planning clinics were for married couples, or those who are about to get married.

- These problems were often acute for *young men* who saw services as run by and for women.

- GPs receive a fee from the Department of Health for providing contraceptive treatment to women, but not men. So there is no financial incentive for GP practices to provide for better sexual health for men (and their sexual partners) through the provision of advice, counselling and condoms.

- In many cases, the Unit heard of youth workers who provided condoms informally to teenagers, where they were unable to get them from other sources.

(iii) Inconsistency in using contraception

7.9 Having the confidence and discipline to use contraception can be another struggle. The Unit heard tales of young women who carried condoms but did not want to produce them for fear of seeming calculating or promiscuous; and many young men who don't like them and women who lack the confidence to insist on using them. Generally, many young people seemed to regard contraception as more 'taboo' than sex. Alcohol is another factor: in one study, two-thirds of people who said drink was the reason they had first had intercourse used no contraception.[132]

7.10 Poor skills in talking about sex, negotiating relationships and taking responsibility for the outcomes may be a significant factor in the UK's high rates of teenage pregnancy. Interestingly, one study found that a far higher proportion of Dutch boys – two and a half times as many as their British peers – discuss contraception with their partners before sex.[133] A US study in 1989 found that men often saw contraception as a purely female concern, yet 40 per cent of women said they relied on men to use contraceptives.[134]

(iv) Failure rates

7.11 Teenagers have a high rate of failure from the contraceptives they do use – principally condoms and the Pill. Condoms are 98 per cent effective if used correctly, but young people may not be aware of the importance of following all the instructions; and the Pill has to be taken regularly and on time. Surveys have identified significant gaps in Pill users' knowledge about what to do if a pill is missed. A small-scale study found half of the Pill users in two family planning clinics could not identify any of the factors (such as missing a pill, vomiting and diarrhoea) which decrease the Pill's effectiveness.[135,136]

7.12 In some other countries, teenagers are encouraged to use other contraceptive methods, which may be more reliable:

■ In the United States, about a quarter of teenagers who have had a baby and 5 per cent of those who have not are now using long lasting contraceptives, which are injected or implanted. Researchers believe this may be a factor in falling teenage pregnancy rates in the US.[137]

■ In the Netherlands, the so called 'Double Dutch' method (condoms plus the Pill) has been promoted to protect against both pregnancy and sexually transmitted infections.

7.13 The Unit found little sign that either of these methods is regularly offered to girls in this country, despite the apparent high rate of Pill failure and condom failure in use, and fast rising rates of STIs among young girls.

(v) Emergency contraception: low awareness and poor access

7.14 Emergency contraception is not a substitute for a regular form of contraception and, of course, provides no protection against sexually transmitted infections. Nonetheless, when a regular contraceptive method fails or is missed, access to emergency contraception may provide a last stay against an unwanted pregnancy. Fewer than 5 per cent of women who use emergency contraception within 72 hours of unprotected sex become pregnant.

7.15 Research in 1999 showed 13 per cent of 16–24 year olds have used emergency contraception on one or more occasions and 5 per cent of 16–24 year olds have used it two or more times.[138] But there are still many barriers to access, especially when unprotected sex takes place at weekends, when it is even more difficult to visit a GP or family planning clinic. In a recent survey, fewer than half of 16–25 year olds knew that there was a 72 hour 'window of opportunity' for taking the emergency contraception pill.[139] The persistence in the name 'morning-after pill' does not help. The result of all this can be seen in a 1990 study that showed 70 per cent of women requesting an abortion would have used emergency contraception instead but did not know how to get it.[140]

7.16 The Unit was told by some groups during its consultation that emergency contraception should be made easier to obtain through making it an over-the-counter medicine available in pharmacies. The issue of whether emergency contraception is suitable for over-the-counter availability is a matter for expert clinical judgement. There are pros and cons. However, the first step is clearly to provide better access to contraception generally, but the Department of Health will keep this under review.

7.17 The boxes in Chapter 10 detail projects visited by the Unit which show promise in tackling the problems set out in this chapter.

8. WHAT HAPPENS TO PREGNANT TEENAGERS?

Three-quarters of teenage pregnancies are unplanned. So decisions about the future are often made at a time of great strain for newly pregnant teenagers. Abortion is more common among young women who see themselves as having prospects that might be endangered by pregnancy; adoption is rare. Support and advice on the options at this time is often haphazard, and there is little provision by professionals for co-ordinated help that will enable teenagers to make an informed choice about the future, and plan for their well-being and that of the child.

"I want to tell my mum, but I can't."

"I've just found out I'm pregnant. My mum gave me three days to decide on an abortion. When I told her I wanted to keep it, she threw me out. But I want to go back home. I miss her."

"My dad threw my sister out when she got pregnant. He's hit her before. I'm so scared I think I'm going to run away."

"I'm 15 tomorrow. I'm pregnant. The doctor told me I should have an abortion. My mum told me to get out and let social services put me in care. I just want to go home."

"I can't deny I was a bit disappointed. She's extremely bright, extremely beautiful and beautiful on the inside too. I wanted more for her out of life. I didn't think she was ready. She's very young."

"I was horrified. She was so young and we wanted her to have a bit of a career before she settled down."

Finding out you're pregnant

8.1 Teenagers are often very late in getting their pregnancy confirmed. For some, this may be because they are not expecting to get pregnant, or have irregular periods or don't keep track of them. Others may fear disapproval or lack of privacy; worry that they will be pressured into an abortion; or are simply 'in denial'.[141] The Unit also heard many stories of young girls carrying their baby to almost full term without seeking help from any adult. A 1979 study found that:[142]

■ a quarter of teenage mothers first consulted their GPs when they were more than three months pregnant; and

■ nearly a fifth had not had their first ante-natal visit until after the 20th week.

Reactions

8.2 A Policy Studies Institute (PSI) study in 1998 found that in the majority of cases, the teenage parent's first concern on discovering they were pregnant was how to tell their parents.[143]

8.3 Analysis by ChildLine of the calls they receive about pregnancy also showed "telling parents" as young people's top concern.[144] Some expressed real fear of being thrown out once their parents found out, or said they would have to run away from home. Overall, of the 3,551 people who told ChildLine whether they had told anyone about being pregnant in 1997–1998:

■ 1,523 had told a friend;

■ only 336 had yet told parents;

■ 301 had told no-one at all and the rest had confided in other family members or adults in the wider community.

8.4 The PSI survey found there was often a more positive reaction to news of the pregnancy from the father of the baby, whereas parents of teenage parents in the same study were disappointed or upset at the news; some were aware of the loss of youth and freedom that becoming a teenage parent entails and had hoped their children would avoid it.[145]

Advice and support

8.5 For the 75 per cent of teenagers who did not plan their pregnancy, the news that they are pregnant will be traumatic. But they need to make, and make quickly, some crucial decisions:

■ Whether to have an abortion or give up the baby for adoption.

■ How to cope with the pregnancy if they continue with it.

■ How to start planning for a future with a child.

8.6 There will, at the same time, be added pressure on their education or employment, and quite possibly strains on any relationship.

8.7 Many teenagers told the Unit they felt short changed by the quality and amount of advice and support they were given. There was no clear responsibility amongst the different agencies and professionals for liaison and no single case worker in charge of discussing the options from all angles. This problem affects those who decide to keep the baby as well as those who have an abortion.

8.8 From the Unit's consultation with young people it seemed that access to abortion varied greatly from place to place and from doctor to doctor. In some cases, young women were put off by staff attitudes they saw as disapproving; in other cases they felt that counselling was simply a recitation of medical history and did nothing to address the emotional aspects. Teenagers often either relied on their family or friends, or took a decision without any adult support at all. Little opportunity was taken when young women presented for abortion to ensure they were properly equipped with contraception to prevent a repeat abortion.

Adoption

8.9 Adoption was once a very common choice for unmarried women who became pregnant. But over the last 30 years, as **Figure 25** shows, there has been a steady decline in the number of adoptions. This is presumably attributable to:

- wider availability of contraception and abortion;

- the decrease in a social stigma attached to being a lone mother: and

- a reaction against strong pressure for adoption in the past.

8.10 Many young women told the Unit and other researchers that adoption was not an option they were counselled about in pregnancy.

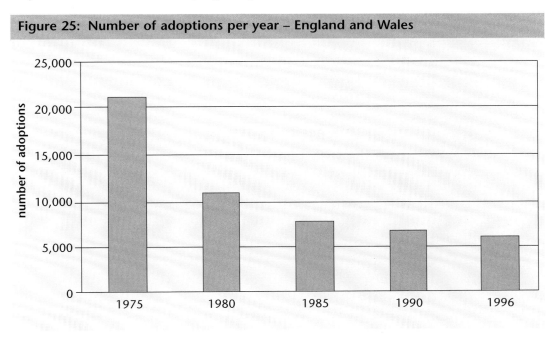

Figure 25: Number of adoptions per year – England and Wales

Source: ONS

8.11 Evidence from the US shows that giving a child up for adoption is more common among teenagers with clear economic or educational aspirations, and from high socio-economic groups.[146,147,148] The Unit has no comparable data on the backgrounds of mothers choosing to give up their child for adoption in this country, but in consultations the Unit found considerable evidence of antipathy to adoption amongst young women, and as US researchers have found, especially from women in lower socio-economic groups.

8.12 The research evidence on adoption suggests that the great majority of young children in adoptive families do well, and many, very well.[149]

8.13 Literature based on the stories of women who gave up their babies for adoption in the 1950s and 1960s suggests that some mothers who give up their children are significantly more prone to depression than others.[150] The quality of counselling they received and the way the adoption was handled are not known but are likely to be relevant to the outcome. Fear of depression appears in what many young women told the Unit:

"Adoption? No way! I've read too many stories about children being mistreated. I'd never give a child up for adoption."

"I never considered adoption. I wouldn't go through all that to give her away."

"I wouldn't be able to live with myself knowing someone else had my baby."

8.14 In August 1998, the Department of Health required local authorities to introduce monitoring systems to prevent children needing adoption from drifting into the care system. Grants are available to local authorities to help them improve their adoption services.

Abortion

■ Amongst under 16s, just over half of all pregnancies are terminated. This ratio has changed little since the mid 1970s.[151]

■ Over a third of conceptions to under 20s end in abortion, and this figure is rising.[152]

■ One in ten 16–19 year olds who have had an abortion had one before, and 2 per cent have had both an abortion and a birth.[153]

■ Pregnant teenagers are also one and a half times more likely than women in their 20s to have an abortion at 13 weeks or later.[154]

8.15 The proportion of abortions paid for by the NHS has increased considerably in the last decade. In 1997, it purchased around three-quarters of the abortions to residents of England and Wales.[155]

8.16 There is considerable variation between health authorities in access to NHS abortions. Some pay for more than 90 per cent carried out under the 1967 Abortion Act, whilst others pay for only around half,[156] but there appears to be little correlation between areas with low NHS payment proportion and those with low use of abortion.

8.17 A greater influence seems to be young women's perceptions of their future prospects. Those who have higher education aspirations are more likely to have abortions than their peers, and students tend to have more abortions than non-students.[157] **Figure 26**, which illustrates the 10 health authorities outside London with the highest and lowest ratio of abortions, shows a trend to a higher ratio of abortions in more prosperous areas.

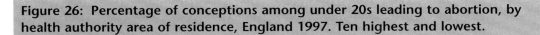

Figure 26: Percentage of conceptions among under 20s leading to abortion, by health authority area of residence, England 1997. Ten highest and lowest.

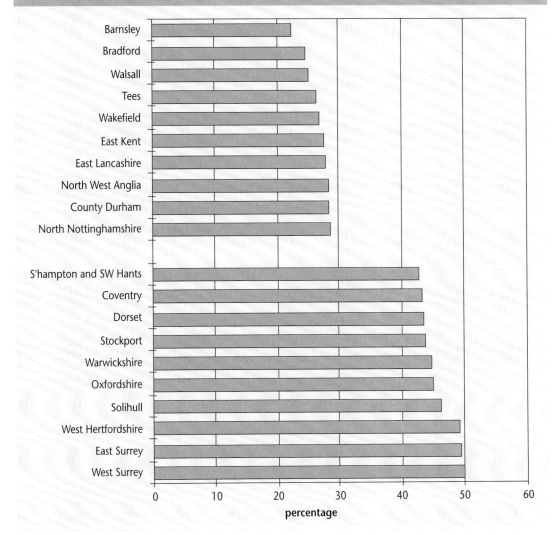

Source: ONS. Figures omit London health authorities – where rates may be affected by a range of factors including the presence of large teaching hospitals and high numbers of abortions to non-resident women.

8.18 In the Unit's consultations young people in more deprived areas appeared to disapprove strongly of abortion, to think it would only be considered by those from more privileged areas who had something to lose, or to feel that if they had an abortion they would be stigmatised by others. The following extracts from discussions with one group of teenage girls are fairly representative:

"I don't agree with abortion – I couldn't do it."

"My mum wouldn't sign the forms for a termination."

"I was too far gone for an abortion."

"My mum offered to adopt the baby."

"I don't know what people feel like when they get an abortion. I've never had one, and never want to have one. But I think in a way, it's a bad way to get rid of a child. Because you have the chance of life, your mum could have just said no. They gave you the chance for life, and you've had a chance to have a life so you should give that baby one chance."

Ante-natal care

8.19 The majority of ante-natal care is provided by midwives (who have a statutory obligation) though this is shared with GPs and consultant obstetricians, depending on local practice. Midwives provide care throughout the pregnancy and usually up to 10 days after the delivery when they hand over to health visitors. They can keep visiting up to 28 days if there is a need – for help with breast-feeding for example.

8.20 But teenage mothers often do less well on ante-natal health than older mothers. There are a number of reasons for this:

- Because the majority of teenage mothers were not planning to get pregnant, they will not have taken preparatory steps that are now common among those planning a baby. For example, a recent survey found that only half of teenage mothers knew folic acid was good for them, compared with over 80 per cent of mothers over 30.[158]

- Because so many present late to doctors, they will not have had early advice on health precautions or got plugged into routines of ante-natal care.

- Statistically, teenage mothers are also disproportionately likely to have some of the risk factors for poor ante-natal health, including poverty and smoking. As **Figure 11** showed, teenage mothers are by far the most likely group of all to smoke before and during pregnancy; nearly two-thirds had smoked before pregnancy and almost a half during it.[159]

8.21 Some of this is reflected in the poor health outcomes for their children, such as low birthweights and higher infant mortality, set out in Chapter 3.

Continuing education

8.22 Attention to ensuring a pregnant teenager continues to receive education is often very weak, and the Unit heard innumerable examples of pregnant girls pushed out of school on grounds of pregnancy or 'health and safety'. This is particularly damaging while educational provision for those out of school remains so poor: an example of a 13 year old receiving only 6 hours education a week from 20 weeks was not at all untypical and for many teenagers this is the beginning of permanent detachment from education. Following the Unit's report on School Exclusion and Truancy,[160] LEAs will be required by 2002 to make available full time education for all children out of school for more than three weeks. New guidance will also be issued in the summer of 1999,[161] with legal force, making clear that pregnancy is not grounds for exclusion, although there is no reason why a pregnant pupil should not go to college or an appropriate off-site unit if that is more suitable.

Looked-after children

8.23 Children in local authority care are particularly vulnerable during pregnancy. In the Unit's consultation, many looked-after children felt they had not received neutral unbiased advice on all the possible options once they knew they were pregnant. Some experienced pressure to have an abortion.

8.24 Research suggests that looked-after young people as a group are more likely than others to be against abortion and most would not consider giving their baby up for adoption. The most likely choice is to carry on with the pregnancy.[162] The National Children's Bureau has estimated that it is twice as common for looked-after young people to want a baby by the age of 20, compared with young people who live with their families.[163]

8.25 Most looked-after mothers told the Unit they had very little education about becoming a parent from school or care and most did not attend the ante-natal and parentcraft classes available locally.

8.26 The boxes in Chapter 10 detail projects visited by the Unit which show promise in tackling the problems set out in this chapter.

9. HOW DO TEENAGERS COPE WITH PARENTHOOD?

> Teenage parents get little of the right support – help back into education, into a job, proper housing and advice on how to be a good parent – and are too often given state support that isolates them from what they need most. This makes it all the more likely that they will remain isolated and on benefit for longer than they need to be. Statistically, the long term prospects for them and their children are poorer than average.

"Although I loved my son I cried for many years after he was born because I lost my independence and childhood, and I resented this. I lost many of my friends through no longer being able to socialise with them. I became very lonely and felt isolated. This life was not glamorous, instead it was lonely and for years I resented this because I wanted to go clubbing and wear nice clothes."

"Soon after he was born, my son developed asthma. It was a frightening experience at 17 years old, watching my son struggle to breathe and not knowing what to do."

"If you could just keep that maternal 'I've got something to love' kind of thing, but it's not like that, it's like a really long day when you are shut indoors watching Teletubbies."

"I tried to go back to school. I wanted to go back, but the school didn't want to know."

"I really want to go back to work. I tried to go to college but they couldn't find me a nursery place. Then they couldn't work out part time hours for me either. I went to my MP, he wrote a letter to my local nursery to get a place for me but it wasn't accepted. I'm doing a lot more than most young mums would do, to get off my arse to try and get work, but it's still out of reach."

"At the time I got pregnant (15), I was in a children's home. I had been in care most of my life. In the April I took two overdoses, I was on solvents, taking drugs and drinking heavily, I was pretty much suicidal. I didn't want to end up on the streets as a junkie, that was the way I was going down. Being pregnant was a reason to live at the time..."

9.1 During consultation, the Unit often heard from teenage parents who said that although they loved their child and were glad they had given birth to them, they had had no idea how hard being a parent would prove to be. At the same time, completing their own education or getting into work seemed unachievable. The benefit system does not encourage teenage mothers back to work or education and lack of child care hinders those who try.

Education, employment and child care

9.2 Many teenage lone parents say that they would like to work and research shows that if they do, this will have a positive long term effect on their children's welfare. Daughters of working lone parents are more likely to do well at school, less likely to be economically disadvantaged and less likely to become lone parents themselves.[164]

9.3 However, many teenage parents face significant barriers to work, the first of which is getting the qualifications necessary to enter the job market.

Education

9.4 Teenage mothers face a range of barriers in getting back into education. Many start with a background of poor experience and attainment at school, and exclusion during pregnancy. On top of this, the interruption of the birth, the stress of coping with a young child or children and the cost and availability of child care are often the final straw.

9.5 At the moment, the system does little to redress these problems, and in practice, local education authorities do not see returning to school as a priority for a young woman with a new baby to care for.

9.6 Specialist Pupil Referral Units for teenage mothers (including special services within a general Pupil Referral Unit) can sometimes offer both child care and the personal attention that motivates and engages young women to return to education. The results can be very positive. General Pupil Referral Units are less suitable, but a common choice.

9.7 Further education colleges are often more suitable and some have crèches, but this is a matter for their choice rather than a right or requirement. There is some central encouragement from the Further Education Funding Council who part-fund child care places in those colleges that apply. This funding is intended to make a contribution to the costs of child care, and as a condition of funds colleges are not allowed to charge users, so must bear the rest of the cost themselves.

9.8 Other avenues which might have been expected to address this need are not specifically designed to target the educational needs of teenage parents:

- the New Deal for Lone Parents, a voluntary programme, focuses on helping lone parents into work or job-related training and does not support child care for education;

- lone teenage parents aged 16 and 17 claiming benefits are unlikely to be automatically referred to the New Deal for Lone Parents because the programme is currently marketed to lone parents with children of school age or above, and teenage parents are unlikely to have children of this age. However, any lone parent on Income Support is welcome to join; and

- the National Childcare Strategy gives priority to the development of out-of-school child care (ie for older children) and teenage parents were not identified as a priority group.

Employment

9.9 Child care continues to be a barrier for those in work. A study in 1996 of lone parent employment in 20 countries showed that the very high costs of child care in the UK, combined with its lack of flexibility created the strongest disincentive to paid work of any of the countries studied.[165]

9.10 Against this background, it is not surprising that few teenage mothers work. A recent study of nearly 100 who had given birth in the preceding three years found that only 11 percent were in paid employment.[166]

9.11 The new Working Families Tax Credit which replaces Family Credit will give greater help to all working lone mothers with child care costs. And in the meantime, the New Deal for Lone Parents can help too by giving advice on in-work benefits.

Benefits

9.12 High proportions of teenage mothers rely on benefit. Nationally:

■ ninety per cent of teenage mothers receive Income Support;

■ teenage mothers are likely to remain on benefit for longer as **Figure 12** in Chapter 3 showed; and

■ teenage mothers are more likely than other lone mothers to rely on benefits alone.[167]

9.13 The benefits available to teenage parents are set out in the box below.

BENEFITS FOR TEENAGE PARENTS

A mother under 16 cannot claim benefit in her own right. However, if her parents are getting Income Support they can claim extra for any grandchildren living with them. Grandparents can also claim Child Benefit.

A mother aged 16 or 17 who is living with her parents can claim Income Support of **£65.05 a week for herself and her child** (figures below are all for mother and child).

A mother aged 16 or 17 living on her own can claim Income Support of **£74.80 a week.**

A mother aged 18 and over can claim Income Support of **£85.50 a week.**

A couple both over 18 with one child can claim Income Support of **£114.75 a week.**

Child Benefit is not paid on top of Income Support.

Those getting Income Support will get help with their rent and council tax.

9.14 Many young parents told the Unit what a struggle it was bringing up a child on these amounts of money. There is little evidence that teenage mothers, especially those no longer in a relationship with the father, receive Child Support in any number. Some grandparents provide financial support but the 1998 PSI study suggested that while some family ties remained strong after news of the pregnancy, others deteriorated severely.[168]

Housing and family

9.15 For many, support from families is in the form of housing. Seven out of ten 15 and 16 year old mothers, and around half of 17 and 18 year olds, stay at home.[169] The rest tend to live in care or social housing (council or housing association properties). One study of young mothers under 20 found that, a year after the birth of their baby, one third were in social housing tenancies with a further third on the waiting list.[170] Studies have shown that homelessness was twice as likely by the age of 33 for teenage mothers as for older ones.[171] The Unit heard from many people that teenage parents were likely to be housed in poor accommodation on large estates often away from family or other support. Teenage parents were six times as likely as other households to live in areas dominated by local authority housing.[172]

9.16 For many young mothers, a flat of their own with a young child is an isolating experience, when they are already isolated from their peers by being a parent.[173] Some specialist housing and models of good practice do offer more adult and peer support, child care, and help with education training and work, but these are not widespread.

Relationships

9.17 For many, lack of parental support is compounded by relationship breakdown. One study found only around a half of teenage mothers were still in a relationship with the father a year after the baby's birth. The rest were usually single and without a steady partner.[174]

9.18 One study followed a group of 174 teenage mothers over 15 years: this found that only 20 per cent of the fathers were still in touch at the end of the period, though for a further 12 per cent there was still contact with an 'early substitute father'.[175]

9.19 More generally, research has shown that all partnerships entered into in the teenage years are much more fragile than later partnerships. Half of all partnerships entered into in the teenage years had broken up by the age of 33 compared with 1 in 5 of those formed in the mid twenties.[176]

Health

9.20 Four out of ten teenage mothers suffer from depression within a year of giving birth – almost double the rate for single women of the same age living at home.[177] Teenage mothers are around twice as likely (8 per cent v 4 per cent) to perceive themselves as being in poor health compared with women who remain childless in their teens.[178] Individuals report a range of stresses including conflict with their own parents, stress of child care on relationships, problems budgeting, going short of food to feed the child; and feeling stigmatised by others. For some, problems are compounded by a second unwanted pregnancy.

Parenting

9.21 In the Unit's visits, some mothers said the arrival of a child was an opportunity to show and receive the unconditional love that they needed, and for some it was a spur to get serious about life, for example by giving up petty crime, or starting to value education more. But most of the teenage mothers the Unit spoke to said that they found parenting far harder than they would have thought possible, and felt ill-prepared for the realities of it.

9.22 A study of 14,000 children born in Avon in 1991–92 produced some evidence to suggest that coping problems were more common among teenagers than older parents. For example, teenage mothers in the study were less likely than average to engage their children in activities such as visits to the library or teaching nursery rhymes, and the children watched more television than their peers. When their babies were 8 months old, the teenage mothers' score on accident prevention was lower than other mothers'.[179] In the population as a whole, accidents, especially poisoning and burns, happen more often to the children of teenage parents than to other children. They are much more likely to be admitted to hospital after an accident or with gastro-enteritis in the first five years of life.[180]

Support

9.23 Many of these problems might be less acute if there were more co-ordination of support for vulnerable young parents. Sure Start will help with some aspects of this as it comes on stream, but at the moment support peters out soon after the birth. Annex 2 gives further details.

9.24 The midwife usually stays in touch for at least the first 10 days, but may visit for up to 28 days if she feels that the mother and baby require this. When the baby is about 10 days old, the health visitor carries out a home visit and first assessment of the family's holistic health needs. Thereafter, the health visitor may have contact with the teenage mother and her baby in a variety of settings, for example in the home, baby clinic or parenting group. Social services will usually only play a role if the mother or child are particularly vulnerable. Voluntary sector groups offer valuable support in some areas, but access to these groups is not spread equally across the country. In the majority of cases, the family is the only source of adult support available.

9.25 Research has shown that young fathers often want to stay in touch with their children and play a proper part in their upbringing.[181] Yet in a small case study on teenage parenthood, focused on a London borough in 1998, it was found that there were no established networks for men or fathering, and that there were few young fathers groups existing in London.[182]

Looked-after young parents

9.26 Teenage mothers in or about to leave care face many of the same sorts of problems as all new teenage mothers – learning to be a parent, finding somewhere to live, getting back into education, finding some child care. They are, however, even less likely to have consistent adult support to back them up and will be more likely to have to move.

9.27 Launching a 16 or 17 year old care leaver with a baby into their own flat with minimal support is a recipe for disaster. But there is a short supply of both foster carers and suitable supported accommodation. Semi-independent units with consistency of staff support and some autonomy are often the best option.

9.28 Once a young woman in care has a baby, the focus of attention often moves from her needs to those of the baby. The chances of the child of a care leaver coming into care themselves are higher than for a non-care leaver.[183] There is a danger that without proper support for both mother and child this can become a self-fulfilling prophecy.

9.29 The boxes in Chapter 10 detail projects visited by the Unit which show promise in tackling the problems set out in this chapter.

10. PROMISING APPROACHES

As part of its consultation, the Unit visited 70 projects in the UK, the Netherlands and the US. The following set of boxes outline some of the schemes visited by the Unit that show promise in:

(i)   sex and relationships education or PSHE;

(ii)   improving access to contraception;

(iii)   supporting teenage parents and their children; or

(iv)   developing local and national initiatives.

Many of the most successful contain elements of all four.

(i)   Sex and relationships education or PSHE

A PAUSE (Added Power And Understanding in Sex Education), UNIVERSITY OF EXETER

The A PAUSE project, established in 1990, is a new approach towards effective schools-based sex education, involving close collaboration between teachers, health professionals and young people trained as peer educators. A PAUSE looks to reduce the increasing medical and social problems associated with some teenage sexual behaviour. Now funded by North and East Devon Health Authority, it is planned that the programme will be delivered to all secondary schools in the Authority's area. The project has also been adopted in North Essex, Teesside and Sandwell.

Aims – the long term goal is to promote the positive aspects of emotional and physical relationships and specifically to: increase tolerance, respect and mutual understanding; enhance knowledge and counteract popular teenage myths; improve effective contraceptive use by teenagers who are already sexually active and provide effective skills to those who wish to resist pressure to become sexually active.

Delivery – elements of the programme are delivered throughout a student's secondary school years. Sessions in Years 7–8 (11–13 years) are taught by teachers, with support materials and training provided by A PAUSE. There are three sessions in Years 9 and 10 (13–15 years), led jointly by teachers and school nurses. Each school receives an annual report, based on data from a student questionnaire in Year 11, which serves as an audit of the school's sex and relationships curriculum.

Peer education – in addition to the teacher and nurse led sessions, in Year 9 A PAUSE presents four peer led sessions. The peer educators are aged 16–19 and their recruitment and training quickly becomes an expected and integral part of the school year. Peer educators have been able to document their involvement in records of achievement and also to relate their experiences to their own studies.

Approach – A PAUSE uses a variety of classroom techniques, including role play, small group discussions and presentations, to encourage young people to consider and discuss issues of sexual health. Such an approach means that those teaching the lesson lower their status in the classroom and raise that of the students. The programme has always recognised that in order to be successful it must make sure that it is actively engaging students' interest.

Impact

The A PAUSE programme is continually evaluated via the Year 11 questionnaire. Results evaluating the overall effects of the school programme, assessed against local and distant control schools, demonstrate that pupils aged 16, who have received the programme, increased their knowledge about sex, contraception and STIs; were less likely to believe that sex is important in relationships; were less likely to be sexually active; were more tolerant of the behaviour of others; and nearly twice as likely to say that sex education was 'OK'.

WEST WALKER PRIMARY SCHOOL, NEWCASTLE

Situated in one of the poorest parts of Newcastle, the school aims to prepare children to become responsible and valued members of society and to take an interest in them as individuals and show genuine caring when they talk about themselves and their lives. The school takes an innovative approach to teaching PSHE, by incorporating it in the literacy hour and other curriculum areas. For example, using well known characters from literature to challenge whether stereotyping is fair, such as 'Stig of the Dump', a character who is outside the 'norm', but who is trustworthy and fair.

Approach – Unit members saw an example of PSHE in the literacy hour when they visited the school. The lesson was about a young girl who had been influenced by her 'friends' to commit a crime. The class studied a piece of text involving a heated conversation between the girl and her parents. Working from the text, the class were asked to think about what motivates people to behave in certain ways, to analyse the attitudes of the mother, the father and the girl herself and to consider the different emotions and feelings of the characters at different points in the discussion.

Role playing – the exercise also included role playing to encourage the children to think about issues from others' points of view. After studying the police statement, one of the children, playing the part of the young girl, was questioned by the rest of the class acting as police officers. The aim is to expose pupils to a range of feelings and experiences.

Visitors – the school encourages members of the local community to visit the school and, through discussions with pupils, allow the young people to gain insights into the feelings of those with whom they may not otherwise come into contact. For example, a group of disabled people recently visited the school and pupils were introduced to sign language.

Community – the school is very actively involved with the local community and a café on the premises is regularly used by parents – helping them to become fully involved in the life of the school. The school plays an important role in encouraging parents to undertake training and further education in their own right. Attached to the school is a community facility in which parents can train to be classroom assistants, crèche workers or to develop their computing skills. The school also employs a worker who is able to discuss parenting issues and family difficulties with parents.

Impact

The school has received excellent OFSTED reports and has been particularly praised for the quality of its PSHE. In addition to strengthening PSHE, the school has increased its SAT scores – helping to treble the scores of its pupils in English, maths and science in the last three years. From being half empty only a few years ago, West Walker now has a waiting list.

SEXWISE TELEPHONE HELPLINE

In many cases, young people say that anonymity is as important to them as confidentiality in seeking advice on sexual health, and there is strong evidence that young men who find it hard to admit ignorance on sexual matters are less averse to using an anonymous telephone line. In March 1995, the Department of Health set up the Sexwise telephone advice line.

Scale – Sexwise has dealt with 2.9 million calls since 1995, but around 32 million calls have been made to the line in that period which did not get through (although many of these will be repeat attempts). Of those who got through, the majority were aged 13–15, and very nearly half were male. This makes it one of the most male friendly forms of sexual health advice available

Service – more than half the calls ask for basic information, and 13 per cent are referred on to other services. Around 40 per cent of callers are provided with specific advice on sex and contraception and 7 per cent receive counselling during their call. Weekends are the busiest periods during term time, and this evens out during school holidays.

Cost – the cost of Sexwise since its inception is around £2.5 million. Running costs are this low partly because there has been no paid publicity for the service since early 1996, so now almost all calls are generated by word of mouth.

Impact
There have been a number of attempts to quantify financial return for early intervention with advice on contraception and sexuality. One of the most conservative estimates is that £11 is saved for every £1 spent on the service, as well as £75,000 which is saved to the NHS for every HIV infection prevented. The continuously high level of unanswered calls, after over a year of no paid publicity, indicates that there is a huge need for such a national service, with well trained counsellors giving impartial information and referral to other services. The success of other telephone lines run by central Government, or voluntary sector ventures such as ChildLine (which also receives many calls on sexual health), shows that such a service has attractions for young people, particularly with its anonymity and easy access.

SPEAKEASY, BELFAST

Speakeasy is a community education project for parents. It takes a community development approach so that parents have ownership of the work, have the chance to influence and shape the programme, and can share their knowledge with other members of the community. Speakeasy aims to encourage parents to provide positive sex education in the home and to offer support and information to parents to take on this role of sex educator.

Approach – the project employs a full time member of staff to work with groups of parents through a series of workshops. All the participants in the programme are mothers. The project worker also runs a series of training courses for professionals in the voluntary, statutory and community sectors.

Goals – to enable parents to develop their own knowledge about sexual health; to explore their personal and cultural attitudes and values towards sex education and to enhance their skills in talking to their children about sex.

Accreditation – the programme has been accredited through the Open College Network (OCN). A number of parents have completed the OCN Level One and a number moved on to OCN Level Two. For many parents, this was their first formal qualification. This provided both a motivation and a tangible output for the parents.

Impact
The project has been independently evaluated and has shown that parents who participated reported that they now understood their role in their children's sex education; that they had overcome their own blocks to discussing sex-related issues; and had learnt information which they could now share with confidence with their children. The parents have also found that their confidence and skills have enabled them to discuss other important issues with their children, including bullying, drugs and peer pressure.

CHOICES, STRABANE

Choices, Strabane is one of four Choices programmes operating in Northern Ireland. Choices is a personal development programme focusing on the sexual health of young women. The programme aims to build the self-esteem, skills and confidence of young women to make informed decisions about their lives and relationships. Within this context, Choices provides participants with the information to build their knowledge and understanding of relationships, sex and contraception. Choices programmes usually consist of between 5 and 12 young women. At the outset, the participants enter a contract – covering issues such as attendance and confidentiality.

Approach – Choices follows a programme which includes topics such as relationships, peer pressure, role models, friendships, communication skills, assertiveness, confidence, sexuality, pregnancy, contraceptives and STIs. A range of resources and approaches are employed through the programme, including videos, games, quizzes and drama. In one exercise, the participants map the leisure opportunities available to them locally. Following this session, the participants in the programme decided to establish their own football team, which now meets weekly.

Location – the group work takes place in informal settings where young people can feel at ease. This has been primarily though youth centres or support agencies. One project uses the facilities of the local heritage centre. The modules used in Choices are accredited through the Open College Network.

Impact
The programme has not yet secured funding for a formal evaluation, though this continues to be sought. However, the group of young women who participated in the programme report greater confidence and assertiveness and a greater degree of control in decision making.

TEENSTARS – LINCOLN MULTICULTURAL MIDDLE SCHOOL, WASHINGTON D.C.

The programme is delivered by the Latin American Youth Center, a local multi-cultural, multi-service community youth organisation. The Teens Trained Around Responsible Sexuality (TEENSTARS) project is a school-based prevention project whose goal is to prevent teenage pregnancy through promotion of abstinence and to establish a comprehensive and integrated approach to the delivery of services to students and their families.

Holistic approach – a combination of sexuality education, social skills enhancement, family activities and a public awareness campaign. The target population is 9–14. The programme uses the 'Sex Can Wait' curriculum for the school-based element. This element is led by an adult facilitator, not a regular classroom teacher.

Core members – typically four or five young people, aged 17–26, assist in the classroom. Around a third of these mentors/assistants have previously taken part in the programme themselves. They also play a part in the regular course of the school day, helping individual pupils with English and maths skills. Many of the core members have gained specific skills and increased their own confidence and self-esteem through working with the project and the majority are now going on to college and employment.

Content – the activities in each five week project are designed to begin to teach young people life skills that can help them to act in their own best interest in all areas of their lives. There are three particular areas of emphasis: Knowing Myself, Relating to Others, and Planning My Future. The emphasis is on addressing many different forms of risk-taking behaviour (such as substance abuse) and making the link between these and unintended pregnancies and STIs. Although the programme does not specifically cover contraception, the Latin American Youth Center does provide a separate clinic for teenagers where they can receive advice and services.

Community base – one of the great strengths of the programme is the existing links that the Youth Center has with the local community. Set up over 30 years ago to support the local ethnic minority communities, the Center has extremely well developed links with local schools, health services, the local radio station and local training services and employers. The Center sees its work in preventing teenage pregnancy as a continuation of its main work of raising self-esteem and self-reliance in the local community.

Impact
Pre and post programme tests have been developed to measure participants' knowledge and attitudes to STIs, sexual activity, abstinence and other topics, and initial results from these tests are encouraging. A six month follow up test will be used to measure further changes in behaviour and attitudes. The Center is hoping to get the Pan-American Health Organisation and George Washington University involved in some further evaluation programmes. Efforts to involve parents in the programme have so far been largely unsuccessful. In recognition of this, the Center is planning new ways of reaching parents, including a programme of active outreach.

PROJECT REACH YOUTH, INC (PRY), BROOKLYN, NEW YORK

PRY was founded in 1968 as a volunteer driven, homework help programme. Since that time the organisation has grown to become a major player in the field of youth leadership development, education and outreach. The organisation has a staff of around 100 and is funded mainly through donations from private foundations.

In 1989, PRY developed a peer education programme which aimed to curb the spread of HIV/AIDS amongst adolescents through raising knowledge and skills and changing attitudes. The result, project SAFE (Speak out on AIDS Facts and Education) now trains over 250 peer educators a year, who in turn reach over 5,000 teenagers in schools, teenage hang-outs and leisure facilities, care homes and juvenile justice facilities. The focus of the project now includes the issues of pregnancy prevention and violence reduction.

Peer educators – are recruited from the communities in which they will be working, often from particularly high-risk populations – those involved in the juvenile justice system and those who are habitually out of school. Before being trained in the specific issues of pregnancy and HIV prevention, the peer educators take part in intensive life-skills training covering issues such as gender roles, diversity, conflict resolution and decision making. Peers make a one year commitment before participating in the programme. In return, their work can count towards school grades and they receive stipends during their time with the project. They also receive formal accreditation as peer educators on completion of their training. Over the course of their participation, peer educators themselves improve their academic outcomes, begin to prepare for college and a career, and take an important leadership role in their community.

Peer video production – in addition to the regular peer education work, a number of young people are working with a local community arts organisation to produce a video on the issue of teenage pregnancy and parenting. At the same time as interviewing their friends, adult members of the community, and medical and social service workers, the teenagers also have the opportunity to explore their personal attitudes to this issue.

Peer Theatre Company – trains advanced peer educators in acting and theatre skills over a series of 12–14 weeks. Together the young people develop a production which includes a series of sketches exploring issues such as peer pressure, dating, relationships, stereotypes and substance abuse, which can then be presented to local young people and other members of the community. After the production, the young people remain in character to field questions and share information with the audience. Initial training for the company came from The NiteStar Program, itself a theatre-centred educational programme for young people, based in the Adoléscent Medicine Division of a large local hospital.

Impact
Evaluation techniques have included pre/post testing, observation and feedback, as well as more formal independent evaluation set up with the help of a local college. Further evaluation is currently under way. Anecdotally, there is no doubt that involvement with the SAFE project has been of great benefit to many of the young people who receive the peer education. Initial results suggest that attitudes and feelings had changed in the peer educators, and that their self-esteem had increased.

BRONX CENTER, PLANNED PARENTHOOD OF NEW YORK CITY, INC

Planned Parenthood of New York City runs sexual health clinics and community based programmes to promote sexual health, prevent teenage pregnancy and to prevent STIs including HIV. They have three promising programmes running in the Bronx and are also beginning to engage local businesses in their campaigns to reduce teenage pregnancy. The Bronx has very high rates of teenage conceptions (168 per thousand), live births (79 per thousand) and abortions (80 per thousand) amongst young women aged 15–19 years (1996 figures). There is also a very high level of joblessness and poverty amongst the mainly African-American and Hispanic population.

Teen Advocates – twenty local young people aged 14–20 have been recruited through church and faith groups, local settlements and community organisations and carefully trained to be peer educators. They use interactive theatre presentations and discussion with the audience to educate about sexual health and pregnancy prevention. The Teen Advocates are exceptional at engaging young people because they are from the community and use teen language and realistic situations in their skits. Performances are in schools, churches and other community bases and have included:

- 'It's up to You Boo' – a skit about abstinence. How do you decide when you are ready to have sex? How do you decide what is right for you? Watch as Sandy makes a difficult decision.

- 'Maybe Baby' – a skit about self-esteem and decision making. A young girl who feels she is lacking in love from family and friends is on the verge of making a decision that will change her life forever.

There has been only one drop out from the group and all the peer advocates report a very positive effect on their own education and achievement. The skits are very well received and enjoyed by audiences and the collation of immediate feedback forms shows a positive effect in developing confidence in dealing with sex and relationships. This group has performed before over 1,000 teenagers in the past year.

Parent Education – the adult role models all come from the same area of the Bronx but have had many different life experiences. Some adults came to the programme as established community leaders, such as PTA presidents and church choir members, while others had histories of addictions or other problems before becoming a part of the programme. They have been recruited through community centres and housing projects and trained to help parents talk to their own children about sexuality and relationships. Participants must complete a rigorous four month training programme on child and adolescent development, birth control, and sexual health, as well as running workshops and special events in the community for other parents and young people. Parents are paid for their participation in the training and for running workshops. This has proved a successful way of engaging members of the community because they understand the challenges and barriers faced by their peers.

Sisters – the staff of the Bronx Center run 12 week groups for the sisters and daughters of teenage mothers. Research indicates that this group is at a four to six-fold risk of becoming pregnant at an early age. The groups discuss growing up and dating, relationships and staying healthy and future plans and decisions.

Impact
Research on the Teen Advocates indicates that their knowledge about sexual health issues has increased dramatically and that their general risk-taking behaviour has also been positively affected by their work. Teenagers who have seen a Teen Advocate workshop report an increased intent to discuss sexual health topics, including birth control and condoms, with their partners and friends following the workshop.

ADOLESCENT SEXUALITY AND PREGNANCY PREVENTION PROGRAMME CHILDREN'S AID SOCIETY, NEW YORK

First set up by Dr Michael Carrera in 1985, the programme works by integrating sexuality and family life education with academic support, career training, health care, counselling, sports and a guarantee of admission to college for every young person (or their parent) who completes the programme. It starts at age 12 and can continue past high school, giving young people compelling alternatives to pregnancy and the tools to achieve their goals. Currently operating in 20 states, the programme is run on a franchise basis, with community leaders who express an interest in developing a programme in their area being provided with the necessary training and support.

Programme content – there are five main activities in each programme, as well as healthcare services:

- education – including homework clubs, intensive tutoring and extra lessons;

- career guidance and job training – including practical, paid, work experience;

- art and drama – developing the creative talents of young people;

- family life and sex education – age appropriate sexuality education; and

- sport – building discipline and self control through individual sports.

All the young people receive free, high quality medical care, access to mental health specialists and general health care advice.

Intensity – the programme operates six days a week, young people arrive straight from school and stay for between two and five hours depending on their age. All the programmes have an active outreach element so those who 'default' on the programme can be quickly encouraged to rejoin.

Participants – those encouraged to join are young people who have all the indicators for future failure – poor school attainment and often families where substance abuse and violence are common. The young people often come from communities where there is little experience of regular employment. Stipends are earned by all young people through the Employment Program (usually every two weeks), on the condition that they open a bank account – a further aid to developing their future.

Location – the Children's Aid Society has developed and helped implement 12 programmes in New York and 33 programmes in other cities in the US. Based in existing community facilities such as youth clubs or leisure centres, all are financed from private donations. Although the programme is similar to 'after-school' clubs, it does not directly involve schools.

Parents – are closely involved with all stages of the programme. Parents must enter into a contract with the programme providers to enable their children to participate. Parents are encouraged to attend at least once a month. There are opportunities for discussions between workers and parents about talking to their children about sexuality, as well as ongoing meetings and personal support. The community workers employed by the programme are fundamental in carrying out this work with parents.

Impact
Two separate evaluations have shown that young people involved in the programme stay in school longer, delay sexual activity longer and attend college at higher rates than their peers. Compared to the US teenage pregnancy average of around 1 in 10, those young women leaving the programme have only a 1 in 25 risk of teenage pregnancy.

INWOOD HOUSE, NEW YORK

Inwood House provides information and support to teenagers in developing the skills and self-esteem they need to resist negative peer pressure and lead independent, productive lives. It runs a range of programmes aimed at preventing teenage pregnancy and providing support for pregnant and parenting teenagers.

Sexuality education – Teen Choice is a comprehensive sexuality education programme, including counselling and parent outreach, teacher training and recreational activities. Project IMPPACT (Inwood House Pregnancy Prevention and Care for Teens) is an abstinence-based education curriculum. Both projects follow a small group mental health model led by masters-level social workers. The groups, which include both boys and girls, meet weekly over a one or two semester period. The goals of the programmes are to assist adolescents in making a healthy transition to adulthood; delay the onset of sexual activity for those who are not yet sexually active and increase positive decision making amongst those who are sexually active; to reduce the incidence of pregnancy and STIs; and to assist parents and their children in communicating with each other about sexuality.

Boys and young men – there are also programmes which work specifically with boys and young men to deter them from becoming teenage fathers with mentoring, counselling and meaningful after-school activities. For teenage fathers there is a Young Fathers programme to provide support in education and finding employment as well as parenting classes to enable the young men to take on their share of parental responsibility.

Supporting parenting teenagers – Inwood House supports pregnant teenagers with a maternity residence for homeless, pregnant teenagers, where they receive pre-natal care, balanced nutrition, educational programmes, and parenting classes, as well as peer to peer mentoring to address the realities of being a teenage parent. The mentors gain self-esteem by serving as positive role models. The Adolescent Parents in Training programme provides a support network, educational and vocational counselling, independent living skills training and parenting classes once the teenagers become mothers. For those teenage mothers in foster care who could still benefit from the guidance of a family environment, Inwood House provides mother/baby foster homes. Child care services are provided to enable mothers to continue their education and training.

Impact
Evaluation of Project IMPPACT looked at a wide range of variables including locus of control, self-esteem, parental relationship and communication, attitudes towards teenage sex and pregnancy and sexual behaviour. In addition to pre and post programme testing, there was a one year follow-up. It found that a small group/mental health programme contributed to attitudinal and behavioural changes consistent with postponing sexual activity and preventing pregnancy. The post-programme testing has found that, although students who were sexually active before the programme began increased their knowledge of sexuality, there had been little comparative change in their attitudes and sexual behaviour. Inwood House is currently engaged in a comparative follow-up evaluation comparing the impact of the Teen Choice comprehensive programmes and the Project IMPPACT abstinence-based programmes.

(ii) Improving access to contraception

THE ZONE YOUTH PROJECT – CORBAN HOUSE SEXUAL HEALTH SESSION, NOTTINGHAM

The Zone Youth Project works with young people in one of the most deprived areas of Nottingham. It offers a wide range of services – career support, drug education, personal skills development and a regular newspaper. The Zone works closely with local faith communities and has been supported by the Church Urban Fund.

Although traditional sexual health services were available in the area, none were specifically targeted at young people and were often held at inappropriate times. The area had one of the highest rates of teenage parenthood in the city. Established in August 1997, the Corban House sexual health session is run in partnership with The Zone, Nottingham Health Authority and Community Health Trust. The project is staffed by two family planning nurses and a receptionist.

Accessibility – the project operates within an ordinary semi-detached house, provided by the local diocese. Sessions are held on Mondays from 3.30pm to 6.15pm. Young people are seen individually, with partners or in small groups. The project is aimed at 12–25 year olds, although the majority of clients are 14–16.

Services – free pregnancy testing and free condoms. Free taxi service to local services for emergency contraception. Information on pregnancy and abortion.

Advice – free, confidential advice on all aspects of sexual health – safer sex, sexuality and contraception, health and general information, as well as referral to Genito-Urinary Medicine clinics, family planning clinics or counselling services.

Support – opportunities to discuss sexual choices, peer pressure and coercion, and relationships. Workers spend a lot of time encouraging and building self-esteem amongst young people. Related issues of drug use, mental health, and family problems can be discussed with trained youth workers.

Outreach – youth workers make links to young people not attending school or youth clubs and make them aware of the services available.

Impact
Between 1997 and 1998 the project provided advice or services to around 400 young people and, unusually, the project has attracted a large number of young men. It is probably too early to say whether there has been a significant impact on pregnancy and sexual health in the area.

THE MAGIC ROUNDABOUT, KINGSTON UPON THAMES

The Magic Roundabout is a self-referral service for young people aged 12–20. Based in a shop front a few minutes from Kingston station, the service is open all day Saturday and late afternoon/early evening during the week. The project has been running for five years and was set up in recognition that an informal counselling service for young people could help to prevent more serious emotional problems in later life. Funded by the Community Health Trust and social services, the project also raises funding independently. The service is run by a part time centre manager and a team of volunteers and is overseen by a management committee which includes representatives from the local community.

Drop-in – an informal advice and information service where young people can come in, have a coffee and talk to volunteer advice workers – who are able to give advice on practical and personal issues and provide onward links to other local services.

Counselling – provided by trained volunteer counsellors. This can cover personal, family, health, education or housing issues.

Sexual Health – operating on a Monday evening and Saturday morning, the service is staffed by doctors, nurses and a receptionist. This provides confidential advice on general sexual health, free supplies, including emergency contraception and referral for abortion.

Outreach – this service works collaboratively with local schools and colleges providing counselling sessions and workshops covering various issues. The service also works with those young people who are excluded from schools or currently being looked after by the local authority.

Impact
Although there has been no formal evaluation of the Magic Roundabout service, the staff hope that in the long term this will impact on the number of unplanned pregnancies.

YOUNG MEN'S CLINIC, WASHINGTON HEIGHTS, NEW YORK

Operating in an economically disadvantaged, mainly Hispanic neighbourhood, of New York City, which also has a significant proportion of new immigrants, the Young Men's Clinic has been in operation since 1987. Developed from an existing family planning clinic, it aims to prevent unintended pregnancy and STIs and to improve the reproductive health of young men and their partners. Operated by Columbia University's Joseph L. Mailman School of Public Health and the Ambulatory Care Network Corporation of New York Presbyterian Hospital, the clinic is part of a broad network of community-based reproductive health clinics and six comprehensive-school-based clinics. Medical services are provided on Monday evening and Friday afternoons in the same clinical space used by the regular family planning programme during the rest of the week. A full time male social worker is based at the family planning clinic on three days of the week, and outstationed to the neighbourhood high school clinic on two days to identify male students at risk for reproductive and other health problems and provide an access point for them to the clinic.

Approach – the Young Men's Clinic reaches out to young men through a variety of means. During the clinic's first couple of years, staff from the clinic co-sponsored summer basketball tournaments, videotaped young men playing basketball in local playgrounds, and offered them the opportunity to watch the video in the clinic – giving the workers the chance to introduce the young men first to sports health and then to more general health issues, including an emphasis on reproductive health. Currently, the clinic social worker reaches out to adolescent and young adult males through a variety of methods which are less labour intensive such as periodic mailings to neighbourhood educational and social service agencies and involvement in community coalitions. The worker conducts brief health education group activities in the family planning clinic waiting room to encourage and enable female partners who are visiting the clinic to refer their male partners to the Young Men's Clinic. The group focuses on testicular cancer amongst young men; asymptomatic chlamydia; communication in relationships and general information about men's health services, including how to make an appointment. Men accompanying their partner for reproductive health visits are engaged in private discussions and then offered appointments to the clinic.

Range of services – a wide range of primary health care services (for example physicals for employment and sports participation) are provided during the clinic's two sessions, with a focus on sexual and reproductive health. Invitations to be screened for STIs are extended to all sexually experienced men. Volunteer medical and public health students, physicians and social work staff assess young men's physical and psycho-social needs. Intensive individual health education including role playing is provided to enable men to increase their use of condoms as well as their support and open communication with sexual partners about contraception and STIs. Short term case management is provided by the social worker for men needing connection with employment, educational, mental health, or other services.

The clinic creates an inviting 'male-friendly' service environment, for example by showing entertainment and sports videos in the waiting room, as well as by conducting at least one health education activity in the waiting room at each session. The clinic tries to maximise 'teachable moments' during which men can increase their reproductive health knowledge, and critically examine their own behaviours as well as the beliefs, attitudes, and values underlying those behaviours. Waiting room group activities encourage men to role play health protective skills such as using a condom and communicating with a sexual partner.

Impact
Formative evaluation of interventions is conducted on a regular basis. For example, a quasi-experimental evaluation of outreach groups working in family planning clinic waiting rooms showed that men were twice as likely to be referred to the Young Men's Clinic by their female partners during the months when targeted groups were offered as compared to months when they were not. As a result of these findings, waiting room activities have become a routine part of the family planning clinic operation. The clinic has been able to show that among the subset of males who in calendar year 1995 made both an initial and follow-up visit, reported condom use at last sexual encounter increased from 32 per cent to 47 per cent, and that there was an increase in the proportion who reported talking with their sexual partner about birth control use, from 43 per cent to 67 per cent.

TEEN TOT CLINIC, UNIVERSITY OF MARYLAND, BALTIMORE

Managed through the Division of Pediatrics and Adolescent Medicine at the University, in addition to medical and nursing staff, the clinic employs a full time masters-level health educator, social worker and nutritionist. The clinic takes a broad psycho-social approach to its work. In addition to contraceptive advice, there is intensive counselling, classes in parenting skills and the development of relationship skills. This includes outings, such as picnics, parties and family fun days, to gain the involvement of grandparents and siblings. The clinic works with many of those who live in the poorest parts of the city, and who suffer from many of the associated problems, including substance abuse, violence and sexual abuse.

Aims – to:

- decrease repeat conceptions to pregnant and parenting teenagers;

- increase immunisations in infants;

- facilitate the young mother's return to education; and

- to improve the parenting skills of the mother.

Access and services – the opening times of the clinic include evenings to enable mothers to attend without missing either their education or employment. Long term injectable contraceptives are increasingly popular. They remove the need for those young women who use the clinic and whose lives are often disorganised to remember to take oral contraception. One such injectable contraceptive, Depo-Provera, is used by over 30 per cent of young women at the clinic.

Outreach – the University also has links with a walk-in clinic in a local shopping mall which increases accessibility for young people. The clinic undertakes very positive outreach to keep in touch with young women who use the service. This includes getting the young woman's permission to contact her via the school, by letter and by telephone – this enables staff to ensure that young women are reminded to re-visit the clinic for further services and advice. Staff are available 24 hours a day.

Teen Tots Dads programme – is an extension of the Teen Tot Clinic. It aims to strengthen the father's role as a parent and to promote safer sexual activity. The programme provides retreats to take the young men out of their normal environment. A specialist worker is employed. Work is done around relationships and building self-esteem. Many of the young men have never received positive fathering themselves and need to develop the understanding and skills to father. The programme helps the young men address issues of education to build their prospects and supports them in finding employment, offers addiction counselling, transportation to the programme and 24 hour access to the facilitator. The programme targets the partners, or ex-partners of those young women who use the regular clinic.

Sisters programme – there is also an outreach programme for the younger sisters of pregnant and parenting teenagers. The main cost for the clinic is providing transportation to bring the younger sisters to the programme. In order to improve health and social outcomes, a clinic is also run for the parents of teenage mothers to help them support both their child and grandchild.

Impact

A control group evaluation for the programme is currently being established. However, there are already a number of positive indicators – the outreach programme has led to 80 per cent of the young women maintaining consistent contraceptive use one year after first coming to the clinic, which compares favourably with only 29 per cent where outreach is not involved. Eighty per cent of the Depo-Provera users were also consistently using condoms. After two years with the clinic less than 12 per cent of mothers have had another child. In addition, there are a number of other general health benefits – 100 per cent of 2 year old children, whose mothers attend the clinic, have been immunized.

(iii) Supporting teenage parents and their children

TEENAGE PREGNANCY SUPPORT GROUP, ST GEORGE'S HOSPITAL, TOOTING

In 1989, a teenage support group was set up by a midwife at St George's Hospital in recognition of the fact that pregnant teenagers often felt anxious about attending clinics whilst older mothers were present. It was thought that many young mothers were missing out on vital pre-natal health checks because of this reluctance. The teenage support group now offers exclusive support, education and continuity of care for pregnant girls under 18, preparing them for the birth of their child and subsequent parenting.

Range of services – clients are referred from general practitioners, are looked after by one consultant and see the same midwife throughout their pregnancy. They are given full pre-natal care, advice on contraception, education and information on parenthood, health and diet, all either individually or as a group. Midwives encourage the families of the young women to become involved and to provide greater support to both the teenagers themselves and the expectant fathers. Parenthood education classes help the teenagers to make informed decisions and to maintain a positive approach towards their pregnancies.

Education – continuity in the young women's education is strongly encouraged. They are given help in making arrangements with school or college tutors for continuing their education. Involvement with education is encouraged until as near the birth as practical.

Access – easy access to morning or afternoon clinics means that teenagers do not have to be absent from school or college to attend. Following the birth of their child, the young women are visited by the same midwife that they first had contact with. Many of those who live locally are also visited at home.

Impact
Although the formal impact of the project is difficult to assess, those working in the group feel that the number of concealed pregnancies and late presenting for pre-natal care in the area has been reduced because of the awareness of the friendly and accessible service that the group provides. In turn, improved obstetric care reduces the danger of fatality or injury to the teenager or their child. The clinic has become an integral part of the Maternity Services, and is well known in the local community.

NEWPIN TEENAGE MUM'S PROJECT, PECKHAM

The project works with young mothers and their children to change the effects of destructive family behaviour and to provide opportunities for positive parenting, to raise levels of self-esteem and increase the educational and employment opportunities available to young mothers. Development work began in 1996 and the project has been open since March 1998. Funding is from the Department of Health, local authority, health authority and health trust. Additional money has been provided by businesses and private trusts.

Parent support group – weekly meetings of young mothers and their children, improving individual skills, advice on looking after both their child and themselves.

Personal development programme – preparation for return to school, further education or employment. The project is responding to concerns about lack of affordable child care on return to education. The local college has agreed to provide a tutor to teach maths and English GCSE to young women, whilst they are at the centre. It is hoped that this service could develop in line with the needs of the young mothers.

Telephone support line – available 24 hours a day, to provide emergency advice and reassurance, and, if necessary, to direct young mothers to appropriate services.

Practical support – help with budgeting and shopping, advice on negotiating the different support systems – housing, social services and benefits.

Impact
Outcomes are difficult to predict as the project is still in its early stages. Over time they expect to be able to show improved mother-child relationships, young mothers moving towards education and employment and reduced involvement with social and mental health services, as well as GPs and health visitors.

CENTREPOINT YOUNG MOTHERS' PROJECT, LEWISHAM

The project has been managed by Centrepoint since June 1993. Its primary aim is to help address the housing needs of local homeless pregnant and parenting teenagers, as well as supporting and advising them around issues such as benefits, parenting, health, education, and training.

Service – there are two full time posts of project manager and project worker based at the unit. Staff provide cover at the project in office hours, Monday to Friday, and the young women have access to staff 24 hours a day via an emergency number. The project worker provides a keywork service to the young women in addition to informal support, and this is used to assess their progress and plan for their resettlement. The residents make good use of the advice service supplied by staff and use staff to advocate on their behalf.

Clients – the majority of the young women who use the project have a history of difficult family backgrounds, and are generally isolated from extended family. There is often little input from the fathers of the children, who also tend to be teenagers themselves. Some of the young women have experience of being in care during some point in their childhood.

Accommodation – there are five bedsits with self-contained kitchen areas, and three bedrooms which share a kitchen. Bathrooms are shared with no more than two other residents. There is a communal lounge with a television and a laundry room with a washer and a drier. Residents have use of the back garden. Residents who have had experience of bed and breakfast accommodation have commented that having their own kitchen, or sharing with a limited number of people, has improved the quality of their day to day lives.

Impact
Generally, the young women who use the project develop good relationships with their peers and act as a source of support for each other, which often continues after they have moved on. The young women are advised that staff support is also available after moving out, and they often update staff on their progress. With a few exceptions, the majority of mothers have settled in to their new homes with no problems.

EDMONDS COURT FOYER, BIRMINGHAM

Open since 1993, Edmonds Court provides 48 fully furnished flats and bedsits to young people, couples and single parents who are in housing need. As well as accommodation, the project provides training, education and employment opportunities – helping residents to gain independence and self-respect. Accommodation is semi-independent and all residents have their own keys. There is no curfew. In addition to a security guard, telephone assistance is available for emergencies. Residents usually stay for around nine months. Resettlement support is available to all residents moving from the foyer into their own home. The foyer is part of the wider St Basil's programme, helping all young people in housing need.

Child care – provided by qualified staff in a registered crèche. Provides flexible child care for residents, enabling them to attend the training programmes being provided on site. The foyer also arranges nursery places off site, for example when a young mother gains a place on a full time college course.

Education and employment – as part of their accommodation agreement, residents are required to participate in a package supporting them into education or employment. The foyer provides careers guidance in partnership with a careers officer and all residents have a tailored action plan. Help is available on searching for jobs, completing application forms and preparing CVs and interview techniques. European Social Fund money has enabled the foyer, in partnership with East Birmingham College, to deliver courses on site, including IT, parentcraft, maths and English GCSEs.

Impact
It may be too soon to assess the long term impact of supported housing schemes such as Edmonds Court. Residents have usually been referred from other projects and are committed to the education and employment package. However, many of those who use the project say that it offers the right combination of housing and support, providing them with the opportunity to do something further with their life. The fact that accommodation is independent, but not isolated, appeals strongly to many of the young mothers.

LANCASTER FARMS YOUNG OFFENDERS INSTITUTION, LANCASTER

Lancaster Farms is one of Britain's newest Young Offenders Institutions (YOIs) and is home to around 500 young men aged between 15–21. They include those on short term remand as well as those who have been sentenced for serious violent crimes. The Prison Service runs a number of parenting and life skills courses in YOIs, amongst which those at Lancaster Farms are considered to be some of the best.

Approach – all the training is presented in a way which is informative, practical and realistic. Their fundamental message is that without parenting training, poor or non-existent parenting skills will persist into the next generation. At the same time, the workers are keen to challenge the negative stereotyping that surrounds young men as fathers, particularly those young men who have spent time in YOIs. The workers who run the courses are both full time lecturers in Lancaster Farms' education department.

Dads R Us – 12 morning and afternoon sessions over six weeks. The content includes cookery and home safety; nutrition and health; being a young parent; role models; responsibilities of fatherhood; legal aspects of parenting such as child maintenance and rights of access; support services and communication. This course is restricted to fathers. On completion, the students gain a certificate from the local college.

Sexual health and parenting – in addition to the Dads R Us programme, there is an 18 session course in Human Development, which is not solely restricted to those who are already fathers. This covers: conception; pregnancy and birth; contraception; role of fathers; child development; health and hygiene and first aid.

Impact

The YOI is working with the Trust for the Study of Adolescence in evaluating the long term success of these projects. Anecdotally, there is no doubt that many of the young men who use this course gain a great deal from it, as one young man said: "I can say that I've learnt a lot from the course, about me, about how I've got where I am. It's given me lots to think about – it's given me some hope in me and in my ability to father my son."

ACCESS TO OPPORTUNITIES (A₂O) – YWCA, NORTHOLT

A$_2$O is a youth and community programme run by the YWCA of Great Britain. The programme is targeting a total of 160 isolated and/or disaffected young women aged 16–19 and offers them a combination of training and work placements. The Northolt project is one of seven YWCA projects taking part in A$_2$O across England.

The A$_2$O project in Northolt began in July 1998 with eight young mothers and one young woman expecting her first child. It is a year long programme and its aims are to increase the participants' self-confidence and self-esteem and their awareness of training and employment opportunities, as well as teaching them new skills and developing existing ones. The programme is run by a part time youth worker and a part time trainer. Accommodation is in temporary units located within the playground area of the local secondary school. The facilities include a communal room where sessions are held, children's playroom, office, small kitchen area and a toilet with baby changing facilities.

Child care – A free crèche is available on site enabling the young mothers to attend the programme while being in close contact with their children should problems arise during the day.

Education and employment – in 1998, the A$_2$O programme included:

- communication skills, including making presentations, listening skills and assertiveness;

- a counselling skills course (essentially to listen well to others, but the course also gave the young mothers the confidence to seek support themselves);

- an IT course;

- work placements;

- completing application forms, CVs and interview techniques; and

- a personal development programme.

Funding – the YWCA provides 55 per cent of the funding, to match 45 per cent from the European Social Fund (ESF) Youthstart initiative. This ESF support is for innovative two year pilot programmes and will cease in early 2000. The YWCA is seeking funding from a range of sources to enable it to continue this type of work.

Impact
Of the eight participants who completed the programme one has secured a university place, five have secured college places and one has been successful in obtaining employment as a result of her work placement. The youth worker reported that there had been a considerable improvement in the personal aspirations, confidence and self-esteem of each of the participants during the year. From a starting point of feeling isolated, unable to cope with the stresses of parenthood, unable to manage their finances or know where to go for help and advice, they now felt they could begin to make reasoned choices about their future in terms of a career or further education.

(iv) Developing local and national initiatives

THE LIVERPOOL PILOT PROJECT

In the early 1980s, Merseyside had one of the highest rates of teenage parenthood in the country. In 1982, the Health Education Council invited Liverpool University's Department of Community Health to develop a pilot project in Liverpool to reduce the incidence of both teenage parenthood and STIs. Identifying an approach widely used in Sweden, which centres on gaining community wide approval for positive changes to the sexual health of young people, the Department developed its proposals via:

Consultation – to establish attitudes among a wide variety of key community representatives, to find out whether there was support for the project, and what the constraining and facilitating factors might be. A wide range of contacts were used, including young people, religious bodies, medical and nursing personnel, youth and community workers, representatives of ethnic minorities and many others.

Workshop – a residential workshop was led by the Family Planning Association, matching the values of participants against the perceived needs of young people. The workshop identified three essential elements of any pilot project: the need for education and training for young people on interpersonal relationships, specific health and general support services aimed at young people and the need for information and media resources.

Support – an important outcome of the workshop was a statement from representatives of the Catholic Church which identified areas of common concern and agreement. This included a willingness to work to deepen personal relationships amongst teenagers, a statement supporting a programme of sex education in local schools and a desire to reduce the number of abortions.

The pilot project proposals were finally rejected by the Health Education Council in 1986.

Impact
But despite the rejection, many of those involved feel that the whole process of consultation and city-wide discussion has in itself been productive; changing the terms of the debate and preparing the ground for new ideas, including subsequent action on teenage conception rates involving the local health authority. In an area of otherwise high rates of conceptions, the rates in Liverpool Health Authority continue on a downward trend.

THE NATIONAL CAMPAIGN TO PREVENT TEEN PREGNANCY, WASHINGTON D.C.

Set up in 1996 in response to President Clinton's challenge in his 1995 State of the Union address that "parents and leaders all across the country.... join together in a national campaign against teen pregnancy to make a difference." A non-profit organisation, the Campaign is funded mainly through private donations. The mission of the Campaign is to prevent teenage pregnancy by supporting values and stimulating actions which are consistent with a pregnancy-free adolescence. The Campaign's goal is to reduce the teenage pregnancy rate by one-third by 2005. It provides concrete assistance to those already working in the field. The Campaign also tries to ease the many disagreements that have frustrated both national and local efforts to address the teenage pregnancy problem in the United States.

Strategy – to achieve their aim, the Campaign has adopted a broad approach:

- Take a strong stand against teenage pregnancy and attract new resources and powerful voices to support this view.

- Enlist the help of the media.

- Support and stimulate state and local action.

- Lead a national discussion on the role of religion, culture and public values in an effort to build common ground.

- Make sure that local community efforts are based on the best available information.

Task Forces – the work of the Campaign is led by four task forces: effective programmes and research; media; religion and public values; state and local action. Task force members have been drawn from many sectors and regions of the country and bring a wide range of experience and points of view. Since January 1999, there has also been a Youth Leadership team, consisting of 26 young people, which advises the Campaign on its work and helps voice the opinions of young people. In addition, cross-party House and Senate Panels play a key role in supporting and encouraging the Campaign's work.

Initiatives – recently included:

- producing a number of well received publications both for parents and teenagers (including the best selling 'Ten Tips for Parents To Help Their Children Avoid Teen Pregnancy') as well as academic research and evaluation papers;

- working with major media organisations such as ABC Television, Black Entertainment Television, Teen People Magazine and other entertainment media to promote teenage pregnancy prevention messages;

- launching a series of Structured Community Dialogues, which bring together community and faith leaders to try to find common ground;

- holding a conference of leaders from 41 states developing media campaigns to help reduce teenage pregnancy;

- making extensive use of new technology – using an extremely professional website to spread good practice, publicise forthcoming events, act as an academic resource and provide down-to-earth practical help to parents and teenagers.

Impact
The teenage pregnancy and birth rates have been declining since the early 1990s, driven in part by reductions in adolescent sexual activity and by increased and more effective use of contraception by sexually active teenagers. The National Campaign hopes to build upon these trends by encouraging all sectors of society – parents, schools, faith communities, health care professionals, community organisations, the media, political leaders and others to work together to reduce further the US teenage pregnancy rate, which remains the highest among industrialised democracies.

11. THE GOVERNMENT'S ACTION PLAN

11.1 Chapters 2 to 9 set out why action is needed to reduce teenage pregnancy.

> **RATIONALE FOR ACTION**
>
> Too many young teenagers are being pressured to have sex rather than really choosing to, are not using contraception, and are, as a result, ending up pregnant or with an STI. Most later regret having started sex too early.
>
> Teenage parenthood is bad for parents and children. Becoming a parent too early involves a greater risk of being poor, unemployed and isolated. The children of teenage parents grow up with the odds stacked against them.
>
> Practical measures can make a difference. These include better information and education; better alternatives to becoming a parent too young.
>
> Preaching is rarely effective. Whether the Government likes it or not, young people decide what they're going to do about sex and contraception. Keeping them in the dark or preaching at them makes it *less* likely they'll make the right decision.

11.2 The report's analysis has also shown the complex set of problems that contribute to the UK's high rates of teenage conceptions and exacerbate the poor outcomes for those who do go on to give birth:

- sex education here often does not equip teenagers with the facts or with the ability to resist pressures;

- access to and knowledge of contraception is patchy;

- there are too many British teenagers who look at their prospects and see no reason not to become parents; and

- not enough is done to get those who become parents back into education and on the road to a job.

11.3 These problems are not insoluble. Chapter 10 shows that there are projects here and abroad that work to combat the problem, and Annex 6 shows that other countries have found that sustained policy approaches yield results.

11.4 The Government needs to learn the lessons of all this. To achieve success there needs to be a credible message to young people and credible policies to back this message up.

11.5 Young people need to be given the facts: the risks of pregnancy and STIs and the consequences of early pregnancy. The messages to young people should be simple and should not preach.

11.6 The policies to underpin this can be summarised under three broad categories:

- **A national campaign** to mobilise every section of the community, including local and central Government, to achieve the agreed goals;

- **Better prevention** of the causes of teenage pregnancy through better education about sex and relationships, clearer messages about contraception, and special attention to at-risk groups. This needs to include young men, who are half of the problem and solution, yet who have often been overlooked;

- **Better support** for pregnant teenagers and teenage parents, to make sure they finish education and learn parenting skills, as well as changes to housing rules so that young parents are not housed in isolated independent tenancies.

11.7 The measures set out below will be funded within departments' existing spending limits over the period of the current Comprehensive Spending Review (until 2002). The ministerial task force will be responsible for securing resources for the strategy in the next spending review.

A national campaign

11.8 No one group – teenagers, parents, schools or Government – can achieve by itself a reduction in teenage pregnancy rates. Tackling teenage pregnancy will mean a concerted effort by local and central Government; Whitehall and town halls and health services will each need new mechanisms to deliver the whole strategy. But it will also need a national effort to change attitudes to teenage sex and parenthood. The national campaign covers England only, but the importance given to tackling the problem is shared by the Scottish, Welsh and Northern Ireland Offices. Together with the new devolved administrations, they will be considering whether the action set out in the report can be applied in their countries.

National campaign		
Action	**Detail**	**Who and when**
1. Establish clear goals	Halve the rate of conceptions among under 18 year olds in England by 2010; and set a firmly established downward trend in the conception rates for under 16s by 2010. Measurements will start from April 1999. Achieve a reduction in the risk of long term social exclusion for teenage parents and their children. This will be measured using the increase in sustained participation by teenage parents in education, employment or training as a key indicator (see Annex 7).	Government adopts these goals and actions to meet them from the date this report is published.
2. National co-ordination	Set up a cross-departmental ministerial task force, chaired by the Minister for Public Health, and an implementation unit in the Department of Health (DH), to oversee implementation.	Set up DH implementation unit September 1999 and task force as soon as possible.
3. Independent advisory group on teenage pregnancy	Set up a national advisory group on teenage pregnancy with an independent chair with a membership incorporating a wide range of views to advise Government and contribute to the national strategy.	Chair and vice chair and members to be appointed by autumn 1999.

National campaign		
Action	**Detail**	**Who and when**
4. Local implementation	The implementation unit in DH will ensure that for each local authority area (LEA and social services boundaries) the local authority and health authority jointly identify a **co-ordinator** who will work through Health Improvement Programmes to: ■ identify the pattern of teenage pregnancy focusing on particular areas, groups, and schools at risk; ■ audit service provision; ■ involve local people and agencies in developing and implementing action plans towards the national goals; ■ link to other relevant local plans and initiatives such as Health and Education Action Zones, Healthy Living Centres, New Deal for Communities Pathfinders, Single Regeneration Budgets, NHS Walk-In Centres, Excellence in Cities and Sure Start.	DH implementation unit by end of 1999. Local co-ordinators to be identified and in place by end of 1999.
	Areas within some Health Action Zones and areas with particularly high rates of teenage pregnancy will, subject to a satisfactory plan be eligible for resources from a Local Implementation Fund (see paragraphs 11.16 and 11.17) to co-ordinate activity to develop integrated and innovative schemes such as peer mentoring and training for parents and for additional advice and contraception.	DH and HMT will explore the scope to increase this fund in the next spending review.
	The implementation unit in DH will issue guidance on this in the autumn of 1999. More detail is in Annex 5.	DH implementation unit autumn 1999.
5. Support co-ordinators	The DH implementation unit through DH regional offices will agree benchmarks for progress with the local co-ordinator by consultation.	Benchmarks to be agreed by September 2000.
	The implementation unit will also provide practical support for local areas on implementation.	DH from December 1999.
6. Monitor progress	The DH implementation unit will identify national benchmarks for the progress of the strategy and the NHS and local authority will produce annual reports for DH based on local authority area.	First reports March 2001.
	The national advisory group on teenage pregnancy will publish an independent report on progress every year to include a summary of national and local progress.	First published report summer 2001.
	The implementation unit will commission better information and research and will evaluate local strategies.	From summer 1999.

National campaign		
Action	**Detail**	**Who and when**
7. Promotion and communication	The Government will co-fund with the private sector fund a national media campaign to reinforce the key messages in this report and will work with the private sector to bolster this.	DH to begin in 1999/2000.

Better education about sex and relationships in schools

11.9 Chapter 5 sets out the weaknesses in the way schools and families educate young people about sex and relationships. Young people must be better prepared so that they can resist the pressure to have sex too young, deal with emotions and relationships, and use contraception if they do have sex. Boys need to be brought into the picture more, and teachers need better support and training.

Better education about sex and relationships in schools		
Action	**Detail**	**Who and when**
8. New guidance on sex education in schools	The Government will issue new and better guidance on sex education in schools, to replace DfEE circular 5/94. The detailed principles are set out in Annex 4. Main elements: ■ **primary schools** must have a policy on sex and relationships education, tailoring what they teach to the age and maturity of the children, but making sure that both boys and girls know about puberty and how a baby is born – as set out in key stage 2 of the national curriculum; ■ **secondary schools** should follow good practice in teaching about relationships and the responsibilities of parenthood as well as sex, focusing on boys as much if not more than girls, involving outsiders such as school nurses, using young people as peer mentors, and being precise about local contraception/advice sources; ■ all schools should **consult parents** and communities regularly and build on evidence of **what works**; ■ **pastoral aspects:** teachers should have more credible guidelines on what to do if they learn a pupil is having sex or planning to do so (see Annex 4). Having a policy that accords with the new guidance will be a condition of membership of the DfEE/DH Healthy Schools Scheme and the resources it attracts.	DfEE to issue draft for external consultation by the end of 1999; PSHE advisory group should be consulted before issue of draft.

Better education about sex and relationships in schools		
Action	**Detail**	**Who and when**
9. Link sex education to a broader framework of personal education	Education about sex and relationships will be supported by a school's wider curriculum on personal social and health education. The Government is publishing a report on PSHE[184] in conjunction with this report which will make the links between education about sex and other related issues such as alcohol, smoking and drugs.	DfEE in conjunction with this report.
10. Teacher training and accreditation in SRE	The Teacher Training Agency (TTA) will review the content and quality of all initial teacher training courses to ensure that pastoral and SRE issues are properly covered for all teachers.	TTA by summer 2000.
	The Teacher Training Agency will produce proposals for the accreditation of specialist SRE teachers.	TTA by summer 2000.
	DfEE will draw together and disseminate good practice guidelines on in-service training for school SRE teachers.	DfEE by summer 2000.
	This will all be reported to the ministerial task force through the DfEE.	DfEE by autumn 2000.
11. Inspection	All OFSTED's inspections (primary, secondary, special, PRUs) will cover the establishment, implementation, and monitoring of SRE policies.	OFSTED to start in autumn 2000.
	OFSTED will survey practice in SRE in a significant number of schools including both good and poor performers and produce a good practice guide on what works for boys and girls for all schools. Report will be seen in draft by ministerial task force and national advisory group.	OFSTED report to be issued to all schools by summer 2001.
	OFSTED will make sure their inspectors are properly trained on SRE and the Chief Inspector will include this in his annual report.	OFSTED from 2000.

Involving parents in prevention

11.10 Chapter 5 demonstrated that children from families that talk about sex are likely to start sex later. But parents in this country are less likely than in some other countries to talk to their children about sex. They are given little help to do this, and many feel they do not know enough about what their children learn at school. This needs to change.

Involving parents in prevention		
Action	**Detail**	**Who and when**
12. Help parents to talk to their children about sex and relationships	DH will commission a national campaign to help parents talk to their sons and daughters about sex.	DH to begin spring 2000.
	DfEE will offer a standard pack of information to parents who withdraw their children from sex education.	DfEE through schools spring 2000.
	The local co-ordinator (see action point 4) will encourage the use of primary and secondary schools and other community centres as a base to support parents in talking to their children.	DH guidance during 2000. Local co-ordinators to report in first annual report in March 2001.
	The DH implementation unit will disseminate good practice for local areas on promising approaches to prevention, including for example, models that are effective for boys, training parents to advise and educate other parents.	DH to begin in 2000.

Effective advice and contraception for young people

11.11 Chapter 7 showed that teenagers in this country are poor users of contraception. While no-one condones under-age sex, the law allows teenagers to have contraceptive advice and treatment in specified circumstances, and they have the right to discuss this confidentially. As part of the Sexual Health Strategy, criteria will be developed for the provision of effective and responsible sexual health services for young people, including advice, counselling and contraceptive services. There will be a new national telephone helpline and a publicity campaign to tell teenagers about their rights to seek help in confidence.

Effective advice and contraception for young people		
Action	**Detail**	**Who and when**
13. Clearer guidance for all health professionals on contraception for under 16s	There will be clearer standardised guidance on the circumstances in which different health professionals may prescribe, supply and administer contraceptives to a person under 16 without the knowledge of their parent or carer. The goal will be to ensure proper implementation and better understanding amongst young people and service providers of the legal framework set out in Chapter 7 of this report. This guidance will set out the counselling that should accompany this provision. This should cover: ■ the case for a discussion with a parent or carer; ■ relationship with partner including possible coercion or abuse (to include the age of the partner and discussion of the law); ■ the arguments for delaying sexual activity; ■ the impact of pregnancy and STIs; and ■ sources of counselling, help and support on issues raised.	DH will draft, discuss with national advisory group and consult externally, and issue by summer 2000.
14. New NHS criteria for effective and responsible youth contraception and advice services	As part of its new Sexual Health Strategy, DH will provide new guidance on the criteria for provision of effective youth contraception and advice services. This will be used to monitor services under the Health Improvement Programme and develop good practice guidance. Special funding for areas with high rates of teenage pregnancy will be available though the local implementation fund as described in action point 4. Improving contraception and sexual health services for young people would also be an eminently suitable focus for a lottery funded Healthy Living Centre. Key principles are that services should be: ■ **accessible** to young people in terms of location, travelling distance, opening hours, including adequate access to emergency contraception, atmosphere, staff quality and training; and reflect the priority young people give to confidentiality; ■ **publicised:** so that all those who may need them know where and when services can be accessed; ■ **joined up:** so staff make the links between eg contraception issues and STIs, or pregnancy testing/abortion and future contraception needs; also link to secondary schools education outside schools and youth services; ■ **effective:** making clear the risks if contraception is not used consistently and what to do if contraception is missed; ■ **open to all:** so boys as well as girls are engaged (may require a review of innovative practices about access to services, eg providing condoms) and services are accessible to ethnic minorities; and ■ **responsible:** offer counselling, particularly for under 16s.	DH to draft guidance, discuss with national advisory group and consult externally and issue by summer 2000.

Effective advice and contraception for young people		
Action	**Detail**	**Who and when**
15. National helpline	DH will build on its work with Sexwise and NHS Direct to provide a nationally available advice line for teenagers to give advice and counselling, and signpost other services. DH has identified resources to pump-prime this and will be exploring further funding with the private sector.	DH, by end of 1999–2000.
16. Get young people to seek advice	DH will fund a national publicity campaign to make young people aware that they have a right to talk to health professionals about sex, relationships and contraception in confidence.	DH will fund campaign to start in 1999–2000 and be repeated as necessary.

Boys and young men

11.12 Young men are half of the problem and the solution. Sex and relationships education in and out of school should bring them more into the picture. Young men also need to be targeted with information about the consequences of sex and fatherhood, including their financial responsibility to support their children. Fathers of children born to teenage mothers will therefore be pursued vigorously by the Child Support Agency to reinforce the message that for this group, regardless of age, they are financially responsible for their children.

Boys and young men		
Action	**Detail**	**Who and when**
17. Publicity	DH will fund a national campaign to ensure that young men are aware of the need for them to be more responsible about contraception, focusing on: ■ the long term impact of an unwanted pregnancy for parents and child; ■ the risks of STIs; and ■ child support responsibilities. DH should commission and distribute to local co-ordinators and NHS providers good practice guidance on how best to target services on young men with sexual health messages through innovative use of media.	DH will fund campaign to start in 1999–2000 and be repeated as necessary. DSS in 1999. DH by 2001.

Boys and young men		
Action	Detail	Who and when
18. Child support	The Child Support Agency will actively pursue the fathers of children born to teenage mothers for early action in calculating how much child support they should pay. As part of the child support reforms to be announced shortly, the DSS will be looking at new ideas for improving the compliance of non-resident parents.	Child Support Agency from summer 1999.
19. Age of consent	The Home Office should consider the views expressed in the Unit's consultation when re-examining the age defence in Section 6 of the Sexual Offences Act 1956.	Home Office in 1999, for public consultation in 2000.

Prevention for groups at special risk

11.13 Those young people most at risk of teenage pregnancy should receive special help and advice. Government action, for example through Education Action Zones, Excellence in Cities and tackling Truancy and School Exclusion, is already helping girls with poor or falling school performance and those missing out on school through truancy and exclusion. The Unit's next report will look at the overall framework for another risk group – 16 and 17 year olds not in education, employment or training. The action points below address the needs of other at risk groups.

Prevention for groups at special risk		
Action	Detail	Who and when
20. Children in care, care leavers and other children in need* (* including disabled children, abused children and sexually exploited children)	Local authority Quality Protects plans (see Annex 2) will contain steps both to help prevent teenage parenthood amongst those children social services are responsible for and better support those who become parents. In-service training for staff will be included. Adequate plans will be a condition of receiving the Childrens' Social Services Grant from 2000.	DH to reflect in guidance during 1999.
	Initial and post-qualifying social work training courses will adequately cover pregnancy prevention and support for teenage parents.	Central Council for Education and Training in Social Work to report to DH by summer 2000. Follow-up will involve its successor body.
	DH and DfEE will produce joint guidance for social workers and youth workers that makes it clear that they can and should direct young people to seek advice and contraception if it appears that they are contemplating sexual activity or are sexually active.	DH and DfEE by summer 2000.
	DH will shortly be publishing a Consultation Paper on 'New Arrangements for 16 and 17 Year Olds Living in and Leaving Care'.[185]	DH 1999.
21. Young offenders	Every Young Offenders Institution will offer sexual health education and parenting classes.	Prison Service to ensure by 2001 that SRE and parenting education are offered in all YOIs.

Prevention for groups at special risk		
Action	**Detail**	**Who and when**
22. Ethnic minority groups	Local co-ordinators should work with local community groups to establish patterns of need for the different ethnic communities and include this in local plans.	Local authority area first report March 2001.
	The implementation unit in DH will audit practice across the country and produce good practice guidance for local areas.	DH to start summer 2000 and ongoing.
	The implementation unit in DH will ensure that better information on ethnic variations in teenage conceptions and parenthood is a priority in its research programme.	DH from 1999.
	The new DH Sexual Health Strategy will ensure that services meet the needs of different ethnic minority groups.	DH from 2000.

Supporting teenage parents

11.14 Chapters 8 and 9 set out how difficult and uncommon it is for teenage parents to finish their education. For many, the damage starts during pregnancy – where support is poor and uncoordinated. Parents under 16 should be required to finish their education and given help with child care to do this. 16 and 17 year old parents should have child care to help them get back into education or training, or to find a job. This will be addressed through some innovative pilots of intensive support in 20 areas as part of Sure Start and a range of measures that will apply nationally.

Education and training for teenage parents		
Action	**Detail**	**Who and when**
23. Getting back into education: Under 16s	Under 16 year old mothers will be required to return to finish full time education and given help with child care to ensure this happens.	DfEE and DH guidance autumn 1999.
	The DfEE draft guidance *Pupil Inclusion* already makes clear that pregnancy is not a reason for exclusion from school.	
	DfEE and DH will issue more detailed guidance on how to support parents or pregnant girls of school age. The principle will be that a period of 18 weeks authorised absence before and after the birth should be allowed, after which any absence will be counted as unauthorised.	DfEE and DH guidance autumn 1999.
	Social services (where the child is a 'child in need') and LEAs will, when the young parents' families cannot help, provide support for mothers of compulsory school age, during pregnancy and after, to make sure the mother can return to full time education, either in school, college or an appropriate unit.	
	Local authorities will report performance to DH.	Local co-ordinators to include in first annual report March 2001.

Education and training for teenage parents

Action	Detail	Who and when
24. Getting back into education: 16 and 17 year olds	16 and 17 year old parents will be able to take part in the Education Maintenance Allowance Pilots from September 1999. Up to £40 a week will be available in 15 pilot areas to those who are living on a low income, or who live in families on a low income. If eligible this will be paid on top of any benefits they are getting. DfEE will explore within the pilot timetable how the study programme and attendance requirements set out in the learning agreement can take account of the particular needs of teenage parents.	DfEE September 1999.
25. Advice for the over 16s claiming benefit	The ONE (formerly Single Work Focused Gateway) pilots will provide teenage mothers who claim social security benefits with an interview with a personal advisor. The personal advisor should discuss options for education, training and work and refer them to appropriate support, training and advice, including the learning gateway for 16–17 year olds, which teenage mothers will be able to take up if they wish.	Employment Services, Benefits Agency and local authorities to pilot from November 1999.
26. Help with child care for 16 and 17 year olds to return to education	The Government will pilot subsidised child care for 16 and 17 year olds whose families cannot help with child care, to allow them to participate in further education or training. This will be piloted over three years in the 20 Sure Start plus areas (see action point 28) and five other areas to assess what type of support is most effective and different ways of delivering support with a view to assessing the viability of a nation-wide scheme by 2003. Young mothers getting Income Support or an Educational Maintenance Allowance will be eligible. The courses need not be directly job related, but should help prepare young mothers to become job ready. In addition, DfEE guidance on Early Years and Child Care Development partnerships will include auditing the needs of teenage	DfEE and HMT to explore the funding in the next spending review. Sure Start Unit in discussion with the DH implementation unit by winter 1999. DfEE guidance for 2000–01.

Supporting teenage parents		
Action	**Detail**	**Who and when**
27. **Advice and support for pregnant under 18s**	In all areas, the local co-ordinator should make sure that in their area professionals and pregnant teenagers have a checklist setting out the services available during pregnancy.	Local co-ordinators by the end of 2000.
	This will list sources of advice on options to keep the baby, adoption or termination. It will also cover counselling, education and training, financial issues, housing and advice on future contraception needs.	DH to issue guidance by autumn 2000.
	The implementation unit in DH will offer guidance on this for local co-ordinators.	
28. **Sure Start plus – personal support for pregnant teenagers and teenage parents under 18**	A new programme to give co-ordinated support for pregnant teenagers and teenage parents under 18 will be piloted over three years in 20 areas which are also covered by Sure Start and Health Action Zones:	Local co-ordinators and Sure Start co-ordinators in consultation with Health Action Zone co-ordinators in 20 nominated areas from April 2000. Areas to be agreed by autumn 1999 (DH will work with Health Action Zone and Sure Start co-ordinators in identifying areas).
	Funding will be found within the Sure Start programme. The programme will have two elements:	
(a) Pregnancy Advisors	Pregnancy Advisors will offer comprehensive advice to enable pregnant teenagers to make a positive choice between continuing with the pregnancy, adoption or abortion. They will also provide advice on future contraception to lessen the chances of a future unplanned pregnancy, and link to education and support. Where adoption or abortion are chosen, expert counselling will be available throughout the process.	
(b) New support package for young parents to help them with housing, health care, parenting skills, education and child care	The service will assess the individual needs of each family including the mother and child and the father, if possible. Their needs may cover health care and contraceptive advice to lessen the chances of a future unplanned pregnancy, child care, housing, managing finances, and parenting skills and may include help from mentors if appropriate.	

Housing

11.15 Chapter 9 showed how often lone teenage parents not living with family are isolated and unsupported. Under 18 teenage parents should not be given lone tenancies for council housing. Those who do not stay at home should be offered supervised semi-independent housing with support instead. Different models for the new form of accommodation will be piloted. DSS will consider how benefit might best support this policy.

Housing for under 18 lone parents		
Action	**Detail**	**Who and when**
29. Social housing: supervised semi-independent housing with support for under 18 lone parents	By 2003, all under 18 teenage lone parents who cannot live with family or partner should be placed in supervised semi-independent housing with support, not in an independent tenancy.	DETR to amend the Code of Guidance on Allocation of Housing and Homelessness to phase this in by 2003.
	Housing authorities will audit provision and need in their areas, and the guidance on the Housing Investment Programme and the Housing Corporation's Approved Development Programme will provide the framework for the capital funding necessary to provide for unmet need.	Audits completed by 2001. DETR and Housing Corporation by 2000.
	In order to kick-start setting up semi-independent supported accommodation, different models will be piloted in a number of areas.	DETR and Housing Corporation summer 1999.
	DETR, DSS and DH will work together to identify necessary revenue funding, taking account of provision already available for care leavers and through 'Supporting People'.	DETR, DH and DSS to explore with HMT the scope to meet any shortfall in revenue funding in the next spending review.
30. Extending same principle to private rented sector through housing benefit	DSS will consider how benefit might best support the policy that 16–17 year old lone parents should be housed in semi-independent adult-supervised accommodation.	DSS by autumn 1999.

Funding the package of measures

11.16 Resources to fund the package have been found from within existing departmental programmes for the period of the current spending review up to 2002. Decisions about funding beyond this date will be made as part of the next spending review.

11.17 A package of around £60 million has been identified for the period to 2002. The Sure Start plus pilots will be funded and evaluated from within the Sure Start programme and are in addition to this. The package includes:

- £26 million for local integrated and innovative programmes in high rate areas (action point 4);

- £0.6 million to support local implementation (action point 4);

- £1.9 million for national co-ordination (action points 2 and 3);

- £3.0 million for research and evaluation (action point 6);

- £7.6 million for publicity to be matched by equivalent private sector funding (action point 7);

- £1.7 million for an enhanced telephone help line to be matched by £1.1 million from private sponsorship (action point 15);

- £2 million to pilot child care to enable 16 and 17 year old parents to return to education or training (action point 26);

- £10 million from the Housing Corporation for bids to pilot different ways of providing supervised semi-independent housing with support (action point 29);

- £0.25 million to provide sex education in young offenders institutions (action point 21); and

- £0.5 million for OFSTED inspections (action point 11).

ANNEX 1: DEFINITIONS

International comparisons

There is no international standard for estimating teenage conception rates. The main factors which preclude ready comparison of conception rates are:

Definition of age

Two different methods are used:

- Age reached during the calendar year of the event (ie abortion or birth). This is the year of the event minus the year of birth. This is the measure used in some European countries.

- Age in full years at the time of the event. This is the age at last birthday and is the measure used in the UK and other English speaking countries.

In order to allow comparisons between the UK and the rest of Europe, Eurostat have produced a set of standard live birth figures for European countries (including the UK). For those countries which calculate live birth rates using the 'age last birthday method', this standardisation has the effect of producing a lower rate.

Comparison cannot be made directly between these standardised figures and those for non-Eurostat countries. **Figures 3** and **10** and the European charts in **Figure 27** use the Eurostat standardisation only; **Figures 2, 17, 18 and 19** use both age last birthday (for US, NZ, Can and Aust) and the Eurostat standardisation (for European countries).

All other figures and the rates in paragraph 1.6 use the 'age last birthday' definition where applicable.

Estimation of teenage conception rates from maternity and abortion data

Maternity rates and abortion rates are calculated separately. Many countries do not aggregate these to produce conception data. It is not possible to use maternity and abortion data from countries which do not estimate conception rates to produce international comparisons. This is because maternities and abortions may relate to conceptions in different years. For example:

- a woman who gives birth at age seventeen and a half will conceive when 16;
- a woman who has an abortion at age seventeen and a half will conceive at age 17.

Population base

Different countries may use different population bases for the calculation of birth or conception rates. The definitions used in England are given below.

England definitions

Conception statistics in England include pregnancies that result in:

■ a maternity – ie one or more live or still births;

■ an abortion – carried out under the Abortion Act 1967.

Conception rates for different age groups use different population bases. The rates used in this report are calculated as follows:

■ Under 20s – total conceptions per 1,000 females aged 15–19;

■ Under 18s – total conceptions per 1,000 females aged 15–17;

■ Under 16s – total conceptions per 1,000 females aged 13–15.

The conception statistics shown for 1997 are provisional. Final figures will be published in Birth Statistics 1998 Series FM1 No 27 in December 1999.

ANNEX 2: GLOSSARY OF GOVERNMENT PROGRAMMES WHICH IMPACT ON TEENAGE PARENTHOOD

Programmes which help prevent teenage parenthood

The UK's first government **strategy on sexual health** was launched earlier this year. Over the next year, the Government will work in partnership with health services, voluntary and community groups and professionals to develop a framework which will set a programme of action on sexual and reproductive health for all health authorities and local authorities in England. The framework will be published next year. (Lead department: Department of Health.)

The NHS will work with local authorities and other local partners to develop a **Health Improvement Programme** (HImP) to be in place by April 1999. The HImP will identify priorities to improve the health and health care of the local population. It may be appropriate to include teenage pregnancies and teenage parenthood as local priorities for action. (Lead department: Department of Health.)

The first wave of 11 **Health Action Zones** (HAZs) was announced in 1998 and a second wave of 15 HAZs in April 1999, targeting special efforts on areas of deprivation and high health need. They aim to reduce health inequalities and modernise services. Each HAZ has identified priorities within its area, which may include measures to prevent teenage parenthood and services for young parents. (Lead department: Department of Health.)

There are a number of new flexibilities which are being introduced into primary care. **Primary Care Groups** will, from April 1999, introduce increased accountability for primary care provision. There may be a need for targeted incentives to improve access for young people to contraceptive advice in primary care through, for example, appropriate training for GPs and their staff. (Lead department: Department of Health.)

Sexwise was established by the Department of Health in March 1995 as part of the Health of the Nation action towards reducing under 16 conception rates. It offers free, confidential telephone advice with the opportunity to talk to a trained adviser about sex and personal relationships and currently receives about 2,500 calls per day. Sexwise has proved very popular which means that a substantial number of callers are unable to get through. (Lead department: Department of Health.)

NHS Direct is a telephone advice line, staffed by nurses, which gives patients advice on how to look after themselves as well as directing them to the right part of the NHS for treatment if they need further medical help. Originally available in three pilot areas, the advice line has now been extended and will be available across the country by the end of 2000. (Lead department: Department of Health.)

The **Quality Protects** programme and other associated initiatives will improve the outcomes for looked-after children in particular and children in need generally and are likely to lead to lower teenage conception rates among this group. The programme will be delivered by local authorities who were asked to submit their action plans to the Department of Health by January 1999. (Lead department: Department of Health.)

The **Healthy Living Centres** initiative was launched at the end of January 1999 by the New Opportunities Fund. This initiative will receive £300 million from Lottery Funds to target the most deprived sections of the population in order to reduce health inequalities and improve the health of the worst-off in society, by 2002. It will be flexible enough to allow for innovative proposals and the different needs of each community, with local key players working in partnership. The type of projects which might be funded could include reproductive health groups and parenting classes. (Lead department: Department of Health.)

Education Action Zones are local clusters of schools – usually a mix of not more than 20 primary, secondary and special schools – working in partnership with the local education authority, parents, businesses, TECs and others. The partnership will encourage innovative approaches to tackling disadvantage and raising standards. (Lead department: Department for Education and Employment.)

Measures which help teenage parents continue with their education

New Start aims to motivate and re-engage 14–17 year olds who have dropped out of learning or who are at risk of doing so. At its heart is a multi-agency partnership working at local level. Young people needing extra help in difficult circumstances, including teenage parents, are being targeted by local partnerships in order to bring them back into learning. Funds have been made available to develop New Start activity throughout the country during 1999–2000. (Lead department: Department for Education and Employment)

As part of the **Excellence in Cities** initiative, to be piloted in six targeted urban areas from September 1999, each secondary school pupil who needs one will have access to a Learning Mentor. The mentors will be based in schools and professionally trained. They will be responsible for making sure that barriers to individuals' learning – in school or outside school – are removed by drawing up individual action plans for each child who needs support and having regular contact with pupils and their families. Learning Mentors will have a specific remit in relation to teenage parents. They will liaise with feeder primary schools to identify vulnerable or disaffected pupils who would benefit from targeted help, as well as helping young mothers to return to school and re-engage in education after the birth of their child. They should act as a support mechanism and link to social services for teenage parents. (Lead department: Department for Education and Employment.)

Pilots for a new **Education Maintenance Allowance (EMA)** will test the effectiveness of a weekly allowance, payable in term time, in increasing participation and achievement in education by 16–19 year olds. The allowance will be available to those who are parents and who live on their own, as well as those who live with low income families. Up to £40 a week will be paid to low income young people in some parts of England to encourage them to stay on in full time education at school or college. The pilots will operate in 15 local education authority areas across the country. If the pilots are successful, then the Government will consider the introduction of EMAs nationally. (Lead department: Department for Education and Employment.)

New national **Student Support** arrangements for post 16s will be introduced from September 1999. Increased access funds will help students with the costs of further education such as transport, books and fees. Colleges will also receive more funding for help with child care costs. (Lead department: Department for Education and Employment.)

Further Education Funding Council provides funding to allow colleges to provide free child care to students – mostly those in receipt of income related benefits. (Lead department: Department for Education and Employment.)

Measures to help teenage parents prepare for work and help with finding work

With resources of £190m, the **New Deal for Lone Parents (NDLP)** offers a personal advisor service delivering a comprehensive package of advice and support on searching for a job, training and child care opportunities tailored to meet the needs of individual lone parents. It is aimed at lone parents whose youngest child is of school age, but parents of younger children are welcome to join. The NDLP can help with child care and travel costs for those who participate in training or attend job interviews, whilst assistance to cover training fees may also be awarded. (Lead departments: Department for Education and Employment, Department of Social Security.)

The **New Deal for Communities (NDC)** is designed to tackle multiple deprivation in the very poorest neighbourhoods. It aims to offer people the opportunity of real and lasting change by improving job prospects; bringing together investment in buildings and investment in people; and through better neighbourhood management and delivery of local services. NDC has resources of £800 million over the next three years to support this programme which aims to bring together local people, community and voluntary organisations, public agencies, local authorities and business in an intensive local focus to tackle the problems inherent to these neighbourhoods. Seventeen local authority districts have been selected as eligible Pathfinder Areas, because their problems are very severe, and are now developing their local programmes. More areas will be included in the programme in later years. (Lead department: Department of the Environment, Transport and the Regions.)

The **New Deal for 18–24 year olds** aims to help young people who have been unemployed and claiming Jobseekers' Allowance for six months or more to find work and to improve their prospects of staying in work. Local partnerships will work together to bring down levels of long term unemployment and to improve the employability of young people in each area. (Lead department: Department for Education and Employment.)

Under **ONE** (formerly Single Work Focused Gateway), people of working age coming into the benefits system will be given support and help in removing barriers to work. The first pilots begin in June 1999. (Lead departments: Department for Education and Employment, Department of Social Security.)

The **Working Families Tax Credit** will be a new tax credit payable to many working families on low or middle incomes and will include a child care tax credit. It will be introduced in October and will replace Family Credit. It will be paid through the wage packet from April 2000. (Lead departments: Department for Education and Employment and Her Majesty's Treasury.)

Under the **National Childcare Strategy**, a Green Paper *Meeting the Child Care Challenge*, published in 1998, set out the Government's plans for good quality child care for all children aged 0–14. The Strategy is being taken forward at local level through the **Early Years Development and Child Care Partnerships**. (Lead department: Department for Education and Employment.)

Measures which support pregnant teenagers and young parents

The Department of Health has provided funding for the National Children's Bureau to develop a self-help guide **Time to Decide**, to support young people in care when making decisions about pregnancy. It includes information about adoption, fostering, abortion, caring for themselves and a new baby, and the further help and support needed to do this. (Lead department: Department of Health.)

A new £540 million programme called **Sure Start** co-ordinates help for families in greatest need to ensure that their children get the best possible start in life. Help will begin with a visit to every local family from an outreach worker within three months of the baby's birth, in addition to other support currently provided. Sure Start will support parents as much as children and may include training for work and help with parenting problems. The first programmes will be up and running by early summer 1999 and by 2002 there will be over 250 Sure Start programmes across England.

A new **National Family and Parenting Institute** will provide the best possible advice and information on all aspects of family life – particularly the role of parents – to government and to groups working to help families across the country. (Lead department: Home Office.)

The **Child Support** scheme supports the principle that parents should take the main responsibility for maintaining their children. Child support can play an important part in helping young people understand the responsibilities of parenthood by spelling out the costs of raising a child. (Lead department: Department of Social Security.)

The **Housing Investment Programme** is the process by which capital funding is allocated to local authorities to build new housing. Local authorities submit their bids to the Government Offices for the Regions who decide how much funding each local authority receives. (Lead department: Department of the Environment, Transport and the Regions.)

Some teenage parents live in **supported accommodation** which provides a range of special services to meet their needs, such as mother and baby hostels where full time help and support may be given. The Government is introducing new arrangements for funding supported accommodation from April 2003 and will allocate a budget to local authorities which will encourage local services to work together to meet clients' needs. (Lead departments: Department of the Environment, Transport and the Regions, Department of Health and Department of Social Security.)

Evaluations of the effect of sex education – overviews

Review	Objective	Key findings
NHS Centre for Reviews and Dissemination (CRD) 1997 Effective Healthcare Bulletin 3(1)	Reviewed systematically the literature on preventing and reducing the adverse effects of unintended teenage pregnancies.	School-based sex education can be effective in reducing teenage pregnancy especially when linked to access to contraceptive services. The most reliable evidence shows that providing sex and contraceptive education within school settings does not lead to an increase in sexual activity or pregnancy rates.
D Kirby, National Campaign to Reduce Teen Pregnancy, 1997 No Easy Answers, Research findings on programs to reduce teenage pregnancy	Reviewed US research on the impact of various school and community-based programmes on teenage pregnancy.	Overwhelming weight of evidence demonstrates that programmes that focus upon sexuality, including sex and AIDS programmes, school-based clinics and condom availability programmes do not increase sexual activity. Studies of a few sex and AIDS programmes have produced credible evidence that they reduced sexual risk-taking behaviour eg by delaying the onset of sex, increasing the use of condoms and other contraception. Attention drawn to limited number of evaluation studies and methodological problems in research designs.
Oakley A, Fullerton D, Holland J, Arnold D, France-Dawson M, Kelley P, McGrellis S, Robertson P Reviews of Effectiveness No 2: Sexual Health Interventions for Young People. London. SSRU. 1994	Reviewed effectiveness of sexual health interventions aimed at young people. Only included randomised, controlled trials in the study base – 12 outcome-based studies from a field of 73. Three studies were based in the UK.	Comparisons between different countries suggested that sexual health information and services for young people promoted good sexual health and were positively linked to avoidance of unwanted teenage pregnancy. The lack of rigorous primary research and evaluation were highlighted. Effective sex education programmes were identified:- Specific programmes improving communication with parents about sex, knowledge and attitudes, and sexual risk behaviour. A specific programme targeting safer sex programmes for teenage runaways.

Evaluations of the effect of sex education – overviews (continued)

Review	Objective	Key findings
Kirby D, Short L, Collins J, Rugg D, Kolbe K, Howard M, Miller B, Sonenstein F and L S Zabin School-based programs to reduce sexual risk behaviors: A review of effectiveness. Public Health Reports, 109(3): 339-360, 1994	Reviewed school-based interventions aimed at reducing sexual risk-taking behaviours in adolescents. Twenty-three peer reviewed studies on school-based programmes were identified by an expert panel which measured the impact of programmes on behaviour. US studies only.	Risk prevention programmes (covering abstinence, contraception, pregnancy, STIs and HIV/AIDS) can be effective in delaying the initiation of intercourse, reducing the number of sexual partners or increasing the use of condoms and other contraceptives, but not all programmes had significant effects on behaviour. The evidence from the studies reviewed indicates that these programmes do not increase sexual activity. Studies based on national surveys provide consistent evidence of no increase in sexual activity amongst older students, but less consistent evidence about their impact amongst younger students. Specific programmes which included instruction about contraception consistently showed either no effect on initiation of intercourse or delayed intercourse.
Grunseit, A and Kippax, S Effects of sex education on young people's sexual behaviour. National Centre for HIV Social Research, Macquarie University, Australia for WHO Global Program on AIDS, 1994	Reviewed studies of the impact of sex education on young people's sexual behaviour.	The review concluded: 'The overwhelming majority of articles reviewed here, despite the variety of methodologies, countries under investigation and year of publication, find no support for the contention that sex education encourages sexual experimentation or increased activity. If any effect is observed, it is in the direction of postponed initiation of sexual intercourse and/or effective use of contraception.' Three studies reporting a delay of sexual activity for those receiving sexuality instruction were identified.
M Baldo, P Aggleton and G Slutkin WHO Global Programme on AIDS paper, presented at the IXth conference on AIDS, Berlin, 1993	Reviewed 18 studies on the effect of sex education in schools. Seven studies evaluated sexual practices (all from US).	In no study was there evidence of sex education leading to earlier or increased sexual activity in the young people exposed to it. Four studies showed sex education led to a delay in the onset of sexual activity. Two studies showed that access to counselling and contraceptive services did not encourage early sexual activity.

Summary of evaluations of specific sex education projects (based on Kirby et al, 1994, Centre for Reviews and Dissemination (CRD), 1997 and Kirby, 1997)

Study	Findings	Comment
Abstinence programmes		Both Kirby (1994)and CRD looked at these studies.
Jorgenson, Potts and Camp, 1993 'Project Taking Charge'	No change in initiation of intercourse.	Kirby: concluded that there was insufficient evidence to determine if school-based programmes focusing just on abstinence delay the onset of intercourse.
Christopher and Roosa Success Express, 1990	No change in initiation of intercourse.	CRD: concluded that these abstinence programmes were not found to have any additional effect compared with the usual sex education programme either on delaying sexual activity or reducing pregnancy. Kirby (1997) reviewed six published studies on abstinence (including the above) and found none to show consistent and
Roosa and Christopher Success Express, 1990	No change in initiation of intercourse.	significant programme effects on either delaying the age of first intercourse or reducing sexual activity. He concluded that the actual impact of these programmes on sexual behaviour is not yet known.

Summary of evaluations of specific sex education projects (based on Kirby et al, 1994, Centre for Reviews and Dissemination (CRD), 1997 and Kirby, 1997) (continued)

Study	Findings	Comment
School-based skills building and factual information on contraception		Kirby (1994) concluded that none of the programmes reviewed significantly increased the onset of intercourse and all included young people of 16 years or younger; some, but not all, the programmes delay sexual initiation; the programmes which had postponing sexual intercourse as their clear goal – Postponing Sexual Involvement and Reducing the Risk – achieved this; some programmes did not have an impact on contraceptive use; other programmes such as Postponing Sexual Involvement, and Reducing the Risk increased contraceptive use for some groups of young people; Schinke-Blythe and AIDS Prevention for Adolescents in School increased contraceptive use among specific groups of students.
Howard and McCabe Postponing Sexual Involvement and Human Sexuality, 1990	Postponed initiation of intercourse. Increased contraceptive use for those sexually inexperienced before the programme started.	
Thomas et al McMaster Teen Program, 1992	No changes in initiation of intercourse, consistent contraceptive use and pregnancy rates.	
Kirby et al Reducing the Risk, 1991	Postponed initiation of intercourse. Increased contraceptive use amongst women and low risk youth. Reduced unprotected intercourse for those sexually inexperienced before the programme started.	Kirby (1997) reviewed 23 sex and HIV education programmes covering both abstinence and contraception (including most of these detailed here). He concluded that the results strongly indicated that sex and HIV education programmes do not increase sexual activity; some, but not all, programmes reduced sexual behaviour eg by delaying the onset of intercourse; some, but not all, programmes increased condom use or contraceptive use more generally.
Schinke, Blythe and Gilcrest, Seattle, 1981	Increased consistent contraceptive use, use at last intercourse and reduced use of inadequate methods.	CRD concluded that programmes combining factual information with skills building had some success in changing young people's sexual behaviour but that omitting guidance on contraceptives and where to access them appeared to reduce effectiveness.
Walker and Vilella-Velez, 1982 Summer Training and Education Program (Step)	No changes in sexual activity, consistent contraceptive use and pregnancy rates.	
Walter and Vaughan AIDS Prevention for Adolescents in School, 1993	Increased consistent condom use.	
Barth RP, Fetro JV, Leland NL, Volkan, K Preventing adolescent pregnancy with social and cognitive skills, J Adolesc Res 1992:7:208-232	Delayed initiation of intercourse.	
Mellanby AR, Phelps FA Crichton NJ, Tripp, JH School Sex Education: an experimental programme with educational and medical benefit. BMJ 311: 414-417, 1995	Increases in knowledge. Relative decrease in sexual activity.	

Summary of evaluations of specific sex education projects (based on Kirby et al, 1994, Centre for Reviews and Dissemination (CRD), 1997 and Kirby, 1997) (continued)

Study	Findings	Comment
School-based programmes linked with contraceptive services		
Vincent et al, School and community program for sexual risk reduction amongst teens, 1987	Pregnancy rates reduced.	Kirby (1994) commented that the Self Center project led to a decrease in pregnancy rates for two years in contrast to a large increase in pregnancy rates in comparison schools. The South Carolina community project, which involved teachers, administrators, community leaders, peer counsellors, and school nurses, produced a significant decline in the pregnancy rates of the 14–17 year olds. After parts of the programme ended, pregnancy rates returned to pre-programme levels.
Zabin et al Self Center, 1986	Initiation of intercourse amongst females postponed. Increased contraceptive use amongst young men and women. Pregnancy rates reduced.	CRD concluded that school-based services linked with contraceptive services could be effective in increasing contraceptive use and that the community-based programme was effective in reducing pregnancies. When this programme was discontinued, rates returned to pre-programme levels.

ANNEX 4: GUIDANCE TO PRIMARY AND SECONDARY SCHOOLS AND ADVICE FOR TEACHERS

Revision of DfEE circular 5/94

Education Act 1993: Sex Education in Schools

The guidance for *primary schools* should cover:

■ how school governors need to comply with the requirement to have a school policy on SRE and must consult with parents when drawing up the policy. There should be targeted consultation with parents before the transition year about the detailed content of what would be taught;

■ whether and how the school might be used as a base for offering support to parents in talking to their children about sex and relationships and how to link this with what is being taught in school;

■ education about relationships such as friendship and bullying and the importance of self-esteem in the early primary school years;

■ the importance of age appropriate methods of teaching, and how the developmental differences among children, particularly in the transition year, may require support and training for teachers answering questions that are not best dealt with in front of a whole class and the provision of individual and small group teaching for some children;

■ clear parameters on what children should be taught in the transition year immediately before moving to secondary school – to include bodily changes related to puberty, such as periods, and how a baby is conceived and born (this should be linked to education about relationships); and

■ guidance for schools on what action should be taken if they have concerns about a child's level of sexual awareness or activity, including the help that can be called on from other agencies. This should be linked to the locally agreed child protection procedures.

There will be occasions when a primary school teacher is directly approached by a primary age child who is sexually active or is contemplating sexual activity. The current DfEE circular 5/94 states that the teacher should immediately inform the head, who in turn should ensure that the child's parents are informed.

The new guidance should:

■ make clear that each school should designate a member of staff (this could be the SRE teacher, or other member of staff with pastoral responsibility or on-site health professional) to whom teachers can go with a child who is in, or contemplating, a sexual relationship; and the designated member of staff should make sensitive arrangements, in discussion with the child, to ensure that parents or carers are informed and that child protection concerns are addressed and that, where appropriate, help is provided for the child and family.

For *secondary schools*, the guidance should again stress the importance of consultation with parents. It should also clarify the principles of good practice for content and delivery.

On *content* this would include the need to:

- set sex education within a broader base of self-esteem and responsibility for the consequences of one's actions;

- give young people a clear understanding of the arguments for delaying sexual activity, reasons for having protected sex, and the ways of resisting pressure to have unwanted sex; and

- provide full information about contraception and how it can be accessed, including information about local services; give young people the confidence and skills to judge what kind of relationships they want and put that into practice, avoiding being pressured into unwanted or unprotected sex (this should link with issues of peer pressure and other risk-taking behaviour such as drugs, smoking and alcohol).

On *delivery*, guidance would cover issues such as:

- how to consult parents in advance and help them to build their skills in talking to their children;

- how people other than teachers (school nurse, other health professionals, youth workers, peers, teenage mothers and fathers) can be involved in SRE lessons;

- use of single sex groups, individual sessions and special arrangements for different ethnic and faith groups; boys should be engaged at least as much as girls;

- developing peer education and mentoring; and

- how those who miss SRE lessons can catch up on another occasion, including the need to ensure that it is covered in education for those out of school.

It is desirable that any young person who is having sex or contemplating doing so talks to their parents or carers about it. The law allows health professionals to see and in some circumstances treat young people confidentially, and part of this process includes counselling and discussion about talking to parents. One of the recommendations of this report is that young people should be more generally aware of the law in this area and of local services to which they can go. Good SRE in schools has a role in delivering this information.

Nonetheless, there may be cases where a teacher learns from an under 16 year old that they are having, or are about to have, sex. In these circumstances, schools ought to be in a position to takes steps to ensure that:

- wherever possible, the young person is persuaded to talk to their parent or carer;

- any child protection issues are addressed; and

- that the child has been adequately counselled and informed about contraception.

The guidance should set out a pathway for dealing with this if it happens:

- The teacher who receives the information should refer the case to a designated teacher for child protection.

- This teacher should, with the headteacher, address any child protection concerns, encourage the young person to talk to their parent or carer and refer on to a health professional as necessary.

It is only in the most exceptional cases that schools should be in the position of having to handle such information without parental knowledge, and where younger pupils were involved this would be grounds for serious concern.

Headteachers and governors should monitor the frequency of such cases. If they are frequent, this points to deficiencies in young people's awareness of, or confidence in, sources of confidential medical advice and this should be addressed.

ANNEX 5: LOCAL CO-ORDINATION

What is local co-ordination meant to do?

Local co-ordination should develop a local strategy that would cover not just sex education and health services but also all services for young people at risk of teenage pregnancy. It would be expected to:

- **identify a local profile** of the picture of teenage parenthood, and groups and areas with high rates, in particular focusing on groups that are known to be high risk nationally;

- **conduct an audit of services** to include preventive services, PSHE in schools, advice and contraception and sexual health services, as well as availability of suitable child care provision, housing, education, training and employment opportunities;

- **consult and involve local communities** by establishing **local advisory groups** (to include all the key local stakeholders, including community groups, parents, young people, media, and faith groups) to meet with and advise statutory agencies to promote community involvement and help develop and implement action plans towards the national goals;

- take forward the Government's wider proposals for **PSHE** and link to **Healthy Schools Initiatives**; and

- link to other **local plans** and **initiatives** such as Health Action Zones and Education Action Zones, Healthy Living Centres, New Deal for Communities Pathfinders, Single Regeneration Budgets, new NHS Walk-In Centres, Excellence in Cities and Sure Start.

Who will co-ordinate?

The local authority and the health authority will **jointly** be expected to identify a **named co-ordinator** for the strategy and involve a minimum range of listed agencies (Primary Care Groups, education, health, social services, housing, careers, Early Years Development Partnerships, TECs and further education, Employment Service and Benefits Agency).

What does local mean?

The co-ordinator will work to **local authority boundaries** (LEA and social services boundaries). This would be coterminous with groups such as the Early Years Development and Child Care Partnerships, Youth Offending Teams and the new arrangements for care leavers, where the links are vital.

Benchmarks

The **national goals** will be divided up by local authority boundary and all areas will have a benchmark. There will be consultation with local co-ordinators about the procedures for setting and measuring benchmarks.

Action plans

Health authorities and local authorities in all local authority areas will be required to submit an action plan every year to the Department of Health, agreed and signed by both the local authority and the health authority and other partners. An annual report on the progress of all local authority areas will be published by the Department of Health.

Mechanisms for achieving this

Health authorities will be in the lead and primary care groups and local authorities will be required by the Department of Health to contribute through the **Health Improvement Plans.** This will be managed through the Department of Health and regional health authorities.

For the local authority (LEA and social services boundaries) the vehicle is the **Children's Services Plan.** A new requirement for the local authority **as a whole** to plan for children has been put forward in the White Paper *Modernising Social Services,* to be legislated when an opportunity arises. **The local authority will be required by Department of Health guidance to include specific proposals to reduce the rates of under 18 and under 16 teenage conceptions and to reduce the risk of social exclusion for teenage parents and their children.**

The Children's Services Plan will summarise the Early Years Development and Child Care Plans and the Education Development Plan and other relevant plans.

For **housing authorities** at district level, guidance will be put in place by the Department of the Environment, Transport and the Regions.

Funding

Local authority areas within some Health Action Zones and other areas with particularly high rates of teenage pregnancy will, subject to a satisfactory plan, have access to a local implementation fund to develop integrated and innovative schemes such as peer mentoring and training for parents and for additional advice and contraception.

The implementation unit in the Department of Health will issue guidance on this in the autumn of 1999.

ANNEX 6: INTERNATIONAL

During its research for this report, the Unit reviewed evidence and research from across Western Europe, the US, Canada, New Zealand and Australia, to attempt to determine a pattern in which places have consistently low teenage pregnancy rates, and why. Unit members visited prevention and support projects in the Netherlands and the US, which are listed in Annex 8.

This research included a major study in 1987, sponsored by the Alan Guttmacher Institute, of 37 developed countries which showed that low teenage conception rates in these countries were associated with:

- high GNP per capita;
- low income inequality;
- high urban population;
- high minimum age of marriage without parental consent;
- openness about sex;
- government policy to provide contraception to young, unmarried women; and
- a high proportion of the population born elsewhere.

The figures below give examples of the decline in rates that have been seen across Western Europe, and more recently in the US. All the charts, except for the US, are based on the Eurostat standardised live births definition. Figures for all European countries have been provided by Eurostat. Those from the US are from the Alan Guttmacher Institute.

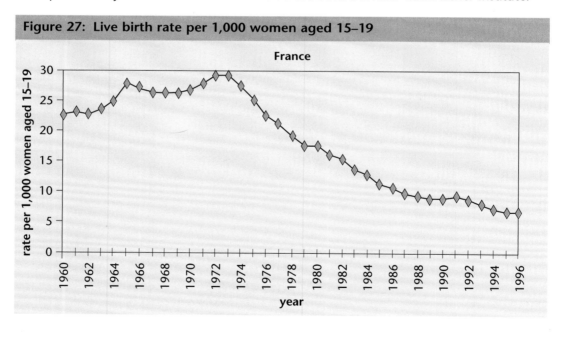

Figure 27: Live birth rate per 1,000 women aged 15–19

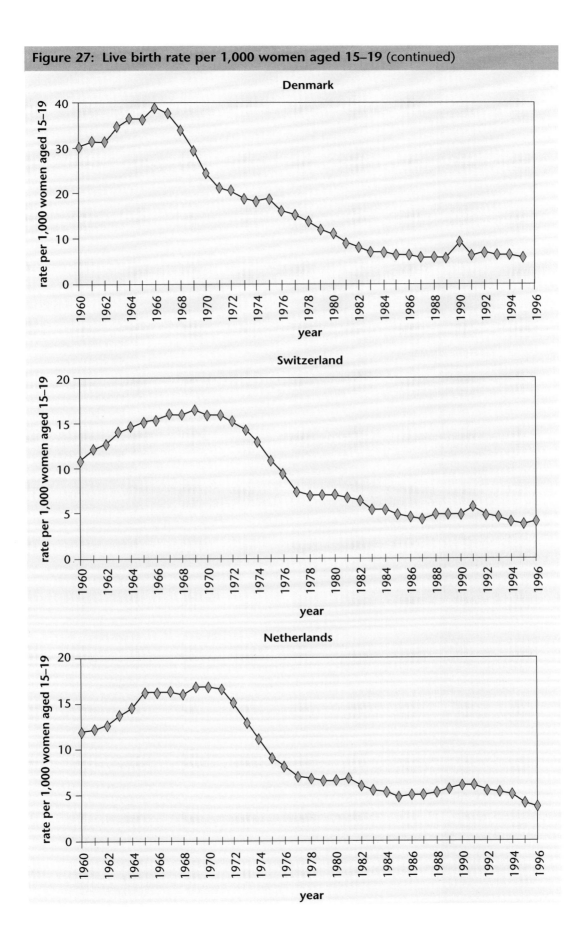

Figure 27: Live birth rate per 1,000 women aged 15–19 (continued)

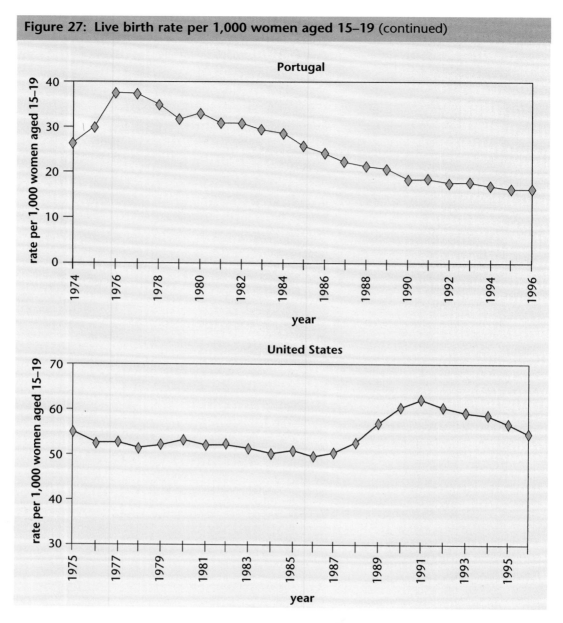

In countries such as the US which have achieved reductions in high rates, there is a debate among researchers about the reasons for the decrease. But there is a growing trend internationally to see teenage pregnancy in the context of poor education and life options of young people, and to tackle that as well as equipping young women with the skills to negotiate and discuss their feelings about sex and contraception.

In the US, for example, the 'Perry Pre-school' programme, which aimed to give early educational support for disadvantaged pre-school children, was found to have a significant effect on reducing the chances of teenage pregnancy a decade later. Although not the formal aim of the scheme, it showed that intervening at a young age to improve the life chances of disadvantaged children is more effective than leaving any intervention until adolescence.

The table on the next page sets out some of the comparisons between law, policy and practice in the UK and 13 other developed countries.

Law, policy and practice

	Age of consent	Contraception		Sex education		
		Provision and availability	Provision for those under age of consent	Mandatory in schools	Content	Right to withdraw child
UK	16 in England and Wales 16 in Scotland 17 in Northern Ireland	Free state provision (except condoms from GPs) through GPs and family planning clinics.	England, Wales and Northern Ireland – see box in Chapter 7. Scotland – the Age of Legal Capacity (Scotland) Act 1991 sets out the criteria. In essence, the consent of a person under 16 is effective if the medical practitioner believes them to be capable of understanding the nature and possible consequences of the treatment.	Yes	Biology (main emphasis), relationships, morality and ethics.	Yes
US	Range varies widely across States from 14–18.	Varies between States and is in the main restricted to the free issue of condoms. There are some private not-for-profit clinics which offer a range of advice and can prescribe a wider range of contraceptive devices but these are not always free.	Varies between States. Title X, the Federal family planning programme, offers a full range of contraceptive services in the clinics which it funds. These are provided without regard to age, and do not require parental consent or notification. Private or State funded clinics may enforce different consent conditions.	No	Varies according to State.	Yes
France	15 (consenting sex not illegal before this age).	Some free samples from family planning (FP) centres, but FP centres poorly distributed and rural areas are ill served. Limited reimbursement for oral contraceptives but situation improving.	Varies across the country. In general, parental permission is required in order to provide under 15s with contraceptives.	Yes	Biology	No

Law, policy and practice (continued)

	Age of consent	Contraception		Sex education			Right to withdraw child
		Provision and availability	Provision for those under age of consent	Mandatory in schools	Content		
Germany	16	Varies geographically. Mostly private FP facilities. Public counselling facilities are poorly used.	Oral contraceptives and emergency contraception are free. Special FP services for young people.	Yes	Biology, personal relationships.		No
Netherlands	16 (sex with 12–15s prosecuted if formal complaint but under 12 prosecution will go ahead even if formal complaint not made).	Near universal coverage by public/private insurance. Contraceptives easily obtainable.	Requests for confidentiality respected. But if attending GP clinic the young person's visit will be recorded on the health insurance documents sent to the parents. Alternative is to visit government funded Rutger Foundation which does not require health insurance cover.	Sex education is not mandatory but Government request that it be given "priority" status.	Biology, relationships, morality and ethics.		No
Switzerland	16	Provision differs according to Canton. Contraception universally available although emergency contraception differs according to Canton.	Medically sanctioned youth services. A few (3) centres offering adolescent out-patient, anonymous services.	Yes	No prescribed nation-wide definition. Practice varies from Canton to Canton.		Yes
Sweden	15, where exploitative 18.	Consultation and advice free of charge. The Pill is subsidised. Condoms are free in youth clinics.	Contraceptive advice and provision available to under 15s. About 130 youth clinics.	Yes	Biology, relationships (main emphasis), morality and ethics.		No

Law, policy and practice (continued)

	Age of consent	Contraception		Sex education		
		Provision and availability	Provision for those under age of consent	Mandatory in schools	Content	Right to withdraw child
Portugal	16 (sex with 12–15s prosecuted if exploitative).	FP services are part of hospitals and mother and child centres where contraceptives are free. Cost of the Pill reimbursed by national insurance system. Charges for IUD, condoms and diaphragms.	Legal for under 16s. Special clinics where age not disclosed.	Yes	Biology	No
Spain	12 (sex with 12–18s prosecuted if exploitative).	Contraceptives only free of charge through special FP centres/campaigns. Problems finding doctor to prescribe Pill free. Pill on sale without prescription at chemists.	There is no legal basis to restrict the provision of contraceptives to those under the age of consent.	Yes	Biology (main emphasis), relationships, morality and ethics.	No
Republic of Ireland	17	Contraceptives sold in private FP clinics, some student union clinics, by GPs, in maternity hospitals and maternity clinics. Provision and availability limited.	Few services provided.	No	Biology, relationships, morality and ethics.	Yes
Denmark	15	Free counselling, no free state provision.	Special FP services for young people.	Yes	Varied	No

Law, policy and practice (continued)

	Age of consent	Contraception		Sex education		Right to withdraw child
		Provision and availability	Provision for those under age of consent	Mandatory in schools	Content	
New Zealand	16	Contraceptives are readily available through GPs, family planning clinics.	No restriction on the supplying of contraceptive advice, or on medical practitioners prescribing contraception to young people under 16 without consent from their parents.	No	Biology, relationships, morality, ethics.	Yes
Australia (Australian Capital Territory)	16	Contraceptives are readily available to all adults through GPs and family planning clinics.	Medical practitioners are able to prescribe contraceptives to those under the age of consent if they are capable of understanding the medical issues and consequences.	Yes	Biology, relationships, contraception, values and decision-making skills.	Yes
Canada	18 Between 14 and 17 can consent to sexual activity where not exploitative.	Many different types of contraception are available – from a variety of sources, including doctors, pharmacies, health centres.	Some variance across Provinces, but generally there is no legal basis to prevent the sale or the prescribing of contraceptives to any individual.	Yes	Biology, contraception, abstinence, healthy sexuality, relationships, STIs.	Yes

	Requirement to be available for work as a condition of getting welfare benefits
UK	When youngest child is 16.
US	Varies across States. For example, Wisconsin requires mothers to work immediately after the child is born. Other States will allow time until the child is weaned. However, the lifetime federal maximum on welfare benefits is five years.
France	All lone parents with a child up to the age of 3 receive a benefit supplement. When the supplement ends, lone parents are encouraged to find work, but can continue to receive welfare benefits.
Germany	Part time when youngest child reaches school age, full time when youngest child is 14.
Netherlands	When youngest child is 5.
Switzerland	No published information available as there are a number of social assistance schemes.
Sweden	Lone parents are required to be available for work, but municipalities must provide child care for children 18 months and over.
Portugal	Those prevented from seeking work because of caring responsibility are exempt from seeking work.
Spain	Must be registered at the National Institute of Employment.
Republic of Ireland	When youngest child is 16 or older, if in full time education.
Denmark	Exempt if local municipality unable to provide child care. Otherwise required to be available for work.
New Zealand	When child is aged between 6 and 13 the lone parent is tested for part time work (15 hours or more). When the eldest child reaches 14, the lone parent will be tested for full time work (30 hours or more).
Australia	When youngest child is 16.
Canada	Age of child for exemption varies between 6 months and 12 years according to Province/Territory.

ANNEX 7: RESEARCH AND INFORMATION PROGRAMME

To provide information for, monitor and evaluate the national strategy for reducing the rate of conceptions amongst under 18s and for reducing the risk of long term social exclusion for teenage parents.

The Department of Health will co-ordinate the programme in partnership with other Government Departments and the HEA, overseen by the ministerial task force.

There are five main strands suggested:

(i)   Better information on variation in teenage conceptions and parenthood

(ii)   Evaluation and monitoring of the national strategy

(iii) Evaluation of pilot programmes of Sure Start plus

(iv)   Technical support for local groups

(v)   Dissemination

(i)   **Better information on variation in teenage conceptions and parenthood**

The national advisory group, the ministerial task force and local partnerships require the best information on the national and local variations in teenage conceptions and births. They need good baseline information on the profile of young parents and the outcomes for their children. Currently, there are gaps in the available information. For example, those campaigning on the issues of looked-after children and ethnic minority health and exclusion issues have drawn attention to the lack of information about the proportions of teenage conceptions and births which are to children formerly in care and to different ethnic minority groups.

■   The Department of Health will review the collection of information on teenage conceptions and births, assessing whether routine systems across government could be improved and feed into the current ONS review of birth registration data with the aim of improving national and local information on variation.

■   The Department of Health will commission secondary analysis of existing or forthcoming data sets to provide additional information about variation in teenage conceptions and parenthood and their outcomes (for example existing and proposed longitudinal data sets, and cross-sectional surveys such as the new National Survey on Sexual Attitudes and Lifestyles).

(ii)   **Evaluation and monitoring of the national strategy**

The national advisory group, the ministerial task force and local partnerships will require a programme of evaluation and monitoring to assess the progress of the national strategy in meeting its goals.

The Department of Health will commission studies on:

■   the impact of the preventive package of measures on the rates of conception including attitudes, sexual activity, knowledge and communication about sex, use of contraception, use of services; and

- the profile and current outcomes for teenage parents and their children, including participation in training, education, employment, family income, health and housing; and track changes over time as the strategy is implemented to assess and monitor the impact of key interventions.

The Department of Health will also explore the potential for current and planned national and local surveys to contribute information for the baseline and subsequent monitoring of the success of the strategy.

(iii) Evaluation of the pilot programmes of Sure Start plus

The Sure Start Unit will co-ordinate an evaluation of the pilot Sure Start plus programmes in discussion with the Department of Health implementation unit, establishing baseline information and outcomes during and after the three year pilot programmes.

(iv) Technical support for local groups

The Department of Health will commission research for the technical support to local groups to identify and evaluate promising approaches to prevention and good practice, including involving young people. This will focus in particular on identifying and helping high risk groups.

(v) Dissemination

All the research outputs will be made public. The Department of Health will design and implement a dissemination strategy for the different elements of research and information, particularly to enable local co-ordinators to make best use of the available information and to involve young people.

ANNEX 8: ACKNOWLEDGEMENTS

In addition to receiving nearly 700 written responses to the consultation exercise, the Unit also met with many individuals and organisations, including:

ACEA
An Nisa Society
Barnardos
Bartley Green Community
Blackliners
Bliss magazine
British Medical Association
Brook Advisory Centres
Bhupinder Manku
CARE
Catholic Agency for Social Concern
Centre for Sexual Health Research, Southampton University
Centrepoint
ChildLine
Children's Express London Bureau
Community Care for Families
Education Development Centre
fpa
Family Welfare Association
Family & Youth Concern
Fred Naylor
Frontier Centre
Green Pastures School of Ministry
Include
INFORM
Health Education Authority
Jain Academy
Joint Council for Anglo-Caribbean Churches
Keith Davidson
Kente
Kingsway International Christian Centre
Leeds Health Authority
London Brook Advisory Centres
Methodist Association of Youth Clubs
Micah Christian Ministries
Mizz magazine
Monkgate Health Centre
Mothers' Union
Moyenda, Black Families Talking
Muslim Council of Britain
Mushkil Aasaan
NACRO
National Children's Bureau
National Children's Home – Action for Children
National Council of Hindu Temples
National Council for One Parent Families

National Council of Voluntary Child Care Organisations
National Health Service, North West
National Institute of Social Workers
National Stepfamily Association
National Youth Agency
NHS Executive, South West Regional Office
Network of Buddhist Organisations
New Testament Assembly
Parent Network
Parents Against Oral Contraception for Children
Probation Service
Queen's Road Health Centre
Raymede Services for Women
Royal College of Nursing
Sefton Health Authority
Sex Education Forum
Shelter
Social Services Inspectorate
Southern Birmingham Community Health Trust
SPUC
St Martin's Hospital, Bath
Surgit Singh Kalra
The Maternity Alliance
Trust for the Study of Adolescence
University College Hospital, London – Dept. of STDs
Who Cares? Trust
Working with Men
Young Women's Christian Association

In addition to these meetings, Unit members visited around 70 projects and organisations, both in the UK and overseas:

Paquin School for Pregnant & Parenting Teens, Baltimore
Teen Tots Clinic, University of Maryland Medical Centre, Baltimore
Hayesfield School, Bath
Speakeasy Parenting Project, Belfast
'Bout Me Project, Belfast
Loud Mouth Educational Theatre Company, Birmingham
St Basil's Centre and Edmonds Court Foyer, Birmingham
Unit for Schoolgirl Mothers, St Philip's Marsh, Bristol
African Caribbean Contact Centre, Brixton
Torridon Infant and Nursery School, Catford
Cotelands Pupil Referral Unit, Croydon
Directorate of Public Health, Croydon Health Authority, Croydon
Croydon Young Peoples Clinic, Croydon
Young Men's Group, Deptford
A PAUSE, University of Exeter, Exeter
Young Women's Outreach Project, Gateshead
Sexwise, Glasgow
Young Mother's Programme and The Grove Project, Hackney
The Magic Roundabout, Kingston Upon Thames
Young People's Advice Centre, Grove House Mother and Baby Hostel, Ladbroke Grove

HEA Regional Seminars: Lambeth, Southwark and Lewisham Health Authority & City and East London Health Authority; Sandwell Health Authority; Newcastle Health Authority

Lancaster Farms Young Offenders Institution, Lancaster

Let's Talk About Sex Project, Leicester

Centrepoint Young Mothers Project, Lewisham

Lewisham Young Women's Project, Lewisham

NHS Executive, Liverpool

Wirrall Brook Advisory Centre, Liverpool

Archway Leaving Care Project, London

Hammersmith and Fulham Social Services Department, London

Royal Borough of Kensington and Chelsea Social Service Department, London

Ministry of Social Affairs and Employment, the Netherlands

Ministry of Health, Welfare and Sport, the Netherlands

Netherlands Family Council (NGR), the Netherlands

Rutgers Foundation, the Netherlands

Stichting Steady project, the Netherlands

West Walker Primary School, Newcastle

Children's Aid Society, New York

Commonwealth Fund, New York

George Washington High School, New York

Grand Street Head Start Programme, New York

Healthy Steps Programme, Cornell University Medical Centre, New York

Inwood House, New York

Madison Square Garden Boys and Girls Club, the Bronx, New York

NiteStar Program, New York

Planned Parenthood New York Inc, Teen Pregnancy Programme, S Bronx, New York

Project Reach Youth, Brooklyn, New York

Young Men's Clinic, Columbia University & New York Presbyterian Hospital, New York

YWCA Access to Opportunities Project, Northolt

The Strelley Project and Outreach Service, Nottingham

The Shepherd School, Nottingham

NEWPIN Teenage Mothers' Project, Peckham

Haverhill Young People's Outreach Project, Suffolk

Central Youth, Young Person's Advice Centre, Stockport

Choices Project, Strabane

The Teenage Clinic, St George's Hospital, Tooting

St. Michael's Fellowship '52', Tulse Hill

Advocates for Youth, Washington D.C.

American Enterprise Institute for Public Policy Research, Washington D.C.

Child Trends Inc., Washington D.C.

Covenant House, Washington D.C.

Department of Health and Human Services, Office of Adolescent Pregnancy Programmes & Office of Family Planning, Washington D.C.

National Campaign to Prevent Teen Pregnancy, Washington D.C.

TEENSTARS, Lincoln Multicultural Middle School, Washington D.C.

The Latin American Youth Center, Washington D.C.

The Children's Hospital, Washington D.C.

The Mayor's Committee on Reducing Teenage Pregnancies and Out-of-Wedlock Births, Washington D.C.

Teen Life Choices, Ward 7, Washington D.C.

Primary Care Condom Distribution Scheme, York

Easingwold School, Yorkshire

ANNEX 9: END NOTES

1   Office of National Statistics (ONS), 1997 *Birth statistics, Series FM1*, 1998

2   ONS analysis of abortion statistics series, 1997

3   K Wellings, J Wadsworth, A Johnson, J Field et al *Teenage sexuality, fertility and life chances*. A report prepared for the Department of Health using data from the National Survey of Sexual Attitudes and Lifestyles, 1996

4   ONS analysis of birth statistics series, 1997

5   K Wellings et al, op cit, 1996

6   ONS analysis of birth statistics series, 1997

7   B Botting, M Rosato and R Wood, Teenage mothers and the health of their children, *Population Trends*, 93, Autumn 1998

8   B Botting et al, ibid, 1998

9   J Hobcraft *Intergenerational and life-course transmission of social exclusion: Influences of childhood poverty, family disruption and contact with the police*, CASE paper 15, LSE 1998

10   N Biehal et al, *Prepared for living? A survey of young people leaving the care of local authorities*, National Children's Bureau, 1992

11   N Biehal et al, *Moving On*, National Children's Bureau, 1995

12   K Kiernan *Transition to Parenthood: Young mothers, young fathers – associated factors and later life experiences*, Welfare State Programme, Discussion paper WSP/113, LSE, 1995

13   K Kiernan, ibid, 1995

14   Croydon Community Trust, *The Health of Young Mothers in Fieldway and New Addington*, 1994

15   Survey by Include in their response to the Social Exclusion Unit's consultation on teenage parenthood, 1998

16   J Bynner and S Parsons, Young People not in employment, education or training and social exclusion. Analysis of the British Cohort Study 1970 for the Social Exclusion Unit, 1999

17   R T Michael, J H Gagnon, E O Lauman and G Kolat *Sex in America*, Boston, Little Brown and Co, 1994

18   ChildLine response to the Social Exclusion Unit's consultation on teenage parenthood, 1998

19   S Maskey, Teenage Pregnancy: doubts, uncertainties and psychiatric disturbance. *J R Soc Med*, 1991

20   M Zoccolillo and K Rogers, Characteristics and outcome of hospitalized adolescent girls with conduct disorder, *Journal of Am Acad Child Adoles Psychiatry*, 1991

21   J Hobcraft, op cit, 1998

22   HMIP *Thematic Review of Young Prisoners* by HM Chief Inspector of Prisons for England and Wales, 1997

23   T Newborn and G Mair *Working with men*, Russell House, 1996

24   K Kiernan, op cit, 1995

25   R Berthoud et al, analysis of Labour Force Surveys 1985–1995, Institute of Social and Economic Research, Essex University

26   Policy Studies Institute (PSI), *Fourth National Survey of Ethnic Minorities*, 1994, 1997

27   Health Education Authority analysis of Health Education and Lifestyle Surveys, 1993 and 1994

28   Health Education Authority analysis of Health Education and Lifestyle Survey, 1994

29   K Wellings, J Field, A M Johnson, J Wadsworth, *Sexual Behaviour in Britain*. The National Study of Sexual Attitudes and Lifestyles, Penguin, 1994

30   PSI, op cit, 1997

31   T Smith, Influence of socio-economic factors on attaining targets for reducing teenage pregnancies, *BMJ* 14 (1) 1232–5

32   Social Exclusion Unit, *Bringing Britain together: a national strategy for neighbourhood renewal*, The Stationery Office, 1998

33   Department of Health statistical analysis of conception rates by type of area, 1997

34   B Armitage, Variations in fertility between different types of local area, Population Trends 87, 1997

35   H Irvine, T Bradley, M Cupples, M Boohan, The implications of teenage pregnancy and motherhood for primary health care: unresolved issues, *British Journal of General Practice*, 47,323–326, 1997

36   J Russell *Teenage pregnancy*, Churchill Livingstone, 1982

37   M Simms, C Smith, Teenage mothers: late attenders at medical and ante-natal care, *Midwife Health Visitor and Community Nurse*, June 1984 vol 20 192–200

38   K Foster, D Lader, S Cheeseborough *Infant Feeding Survey 1995*, TSO, 1997

39   Foster et al, ibid, 1997

40   K Kiernan, G Mueller, *The Divorced and Who Divorces*, CASE paper 7, LSE 1998

41   I Allen, S Bourke Dowling, *Teenage Mothers: Decisions and outcomes*, Policy Studies Institute, 1998

42   I Allen et al, ibid, 1998

43   S Speak, S Cameron, R Woods, R Gilroy, *Young single mothers: barriers to independent living*, Family Policy Studies Centre, 1995

44   I Allen et al, ibid, 1998

45   Department of Social Security (DSS) analysis of Income Support claimants, 1993–1998. Ninety per cent of teenagers receiving Income Support includes all teenage parents, whatever the age of their child. Figure 12 analysis controls for age of child.

46   B Botting et al, op cit, 1998

47   B Botting et al, ibid, 1998

48   N Dattani, Mortality in children aged under 4, *Health Statistics Quarterly 02*, Office for National Statistics, 1999

49   J Wilson, Maternity Policy. Caroline: a case of a pregnant teenager, *Professional care of mother and child*, Vol 5,5, 139–142, 1995

50   Foster et al, op cit, 1997

51   S Peckham, Preventing unplanned teenage pregnancies, *Public Health*, 1993, 107 125–133

52   J Hobcraft and K Kiernan *Childhood Poverty, Early Motherhood, and Adult Social Exclusion*. Analysis for the Social Exclusion Unit, CASE paper 28, LSE 1999. The analyses of the effects of teenage motherhood and of childhood poverty on adverse adult outcomes are drawn from logistic regression models, which control for both of these factors and for a wide range of other potential childhood factors, including family type, contact with the police, father's and mother's interest in schooling, mother's and father's school leaving age, parental housing tenure, grandfathers' and father's social class, personality attributes (aggression, anxiety, and restlessness), and test scores. For details of these factors see J Hobcraft (1998) CASE paper 15.

53   J Hobcraft and K Kiernan, ibid, 1999

54   J Hobcraft and K Kiernan, ibid, 1999

55   Department of Social Security (DSS) analysis of data from Households Below Average Income Series, 1996/7

56   J Bynner, E Ferri, P Shepherd *Twenty somethings in the 1990s*, Ashgate, 1997

57   K Kiernan, op cit, 1995

58   K Kiernan et al, op cit, 1998

59   K Kiernan, op cit, 1995

60   K Kiernan, op cit, 1995

61   B Botting et al, op cit, 1998

62   K Kiernan et al , op cit, 1998

63   K Wellings et al, op cit, 1996

64   L Clarke, H Joshi, P DiSalvo, J Wright, *Stability and instability in children's family lives: longitudinal evidence from two British Sources*, Centre for Population Studies Research Paper 97-1 City University, London 1997

65   B C Clewell, J Brooks Gunn, A A Benasich, Evaluating child related outcomes of teenage parenting programs *FAMR* 1989; 38:201–209

66   M Simms, C Smith *Teenage mothers and their partners: a survey in England and Wales*, HMSO, 1986

67   S Williams, J Forbes, GM Mellwaine, K Rosenberg, Poverty and teenage pregnancy, *BMJ* 1987; 294:20–21

68   K Kiernan, op cit, 1995

69   I Allen et al, op cit, 1998

70   Health Education Authority analysis of data from surveys on smoking and pregnancy 1994–1998

71   R Kane and K Wellings, *Reducing the rate of teenage conceptions: Data from Europe*, Health Education Authority, London, 1999

72   S Cheesebrough, R Ingham, D Massey, *Reducing the rate of teenage conceptions. An international review of the evidence: USA, Canada, Australia and New Zealand*, Health Education Authority, London, 1999

73   Data is not available from the same source year and, as with live birth figures, is collected in different, and not always consistent, ways. In addition, it is known that women travel outside their own country to seek abortions which are not readily available at home.

74   Health Education Authority *Unintended teenage conceptions, Qualitative research to inform the national programme to reduce the rate of unintended teenage conceptions*, 1998

75   I Allen et al, op cit, 1998

76   I Allen et al, op cit, 1998

77   Department of Environment, Transport and the Regions (DETR) unpublished analysis of data from the Survey of English Housing, 1996/97

78   Social Exclusion Unit, op cit, 1998

79   J Bradshaw et al, *The Employment of lone parents: a comparison of policy in 20 countries*, Family Policy Studies Centre, 1996

80   D Kirby, *No Easy Answers, Research findings on programs to reduce teen pregnancy*. National program for the reduction in teenage pregnancies, 1997

81   R Kane et al, op cit, 1999

82   P Donovan, Falling Teen Pregnancy, Birthrates, What's behind the declines?, *The Guttmacher report on public policy*, Vol. 1, No 5 October 1998. The Alan Guttmacher Institute, 1998

83   K Wellings et al, op cit, 1996

84   K Wellings et al, *The National Survey of Sexual Attitudes and Lifestyles: Teenage Pregnancy*, ESRC Research Results, 1997

85   NHS Centre for Reviews and Dissemination (CRD), *Effective Healthcare Bulletin 3 (1)* Prevention and reducing the adverse effects of unintended teenage pregnancies, University of York, 1997

86   D Kirby, op cit, 1997

87   D Kirby, L Short, J Collins, D Rugg, K Kolbe, M Howard, B Miller, F Sonenstein and L S Zabin, School-based programs to reduce sexual risk behaviors: A review of effectiveness, *Public Health Reports*, 109(3): 339–360, 1994

88   A Grunseit, and S Kippax, Effects of sex education on young people's sexual behaviour. National Centre for HIV Social Research, Macquarie University, Australia for WHO Global Program on AIDS, 1994

89   M Baldo, P Aggleton and G Slutkin, WHO Global Programme on AIDS paper, presented at the IXth conference on AIDS, Berlin, 1993

90   K Wellings et al, op cit, 1996

91   I Allen, *Education in Sex and Personal relationships*, Policy Studies Institute, 1987

92   HEA and National Foundation for Education Research In England and Wales, *Parents, schools and sex education – a compelling case for partnership*, London, HEA, 1994

93   K Wellings et al, op cit, 1996

94   Health Education Authority, *Young People and Health,* HEA, 1999

95   Health Education Authority/Office for National Statistics Omnibus Survey, 1998

96   S Livingstone and M Borrill, *Young People, New Media*, 1999

97   S Prendergast, *This is the time to grow up. Girls experiences of menstruation in school*, Health Promotion Research Trust, 1992

98   Health Education Authority, *Young People and Health*, HEA, 1999

99   Department for Education and Employment communication 1998. OFSTED estimate based on information from Local Education Authority Advisers.

100   Department of Education circular 5/94, Education Act 1993: *Sex Education in Schools*

101   S Clements, R Ingham, N Stone and I Diamond, *Young people's views on sexual health, services and sex education*, results of a survey in a large secondary school. Unpublished report, Centre for Sexual Health, University of Southampton, 1999

102   Health Education Authority, *Unintended teenage conceptions; Qualitative research to inform the national programme to reduce the rate of unintended teenage conceptions*, HEA, 1998

103   C Carrera and R Ingham, *Exploration of the factors that affect the delivery of sex and sexuality education and support in schools – a selective literature review*, Centre for Sexual Health Research, Faculty of Social Sciences, University of Southampton, 1997

104   R Ingham et al, *Exploration of the factors that affect the delivery of sex and sexuality education and support in schools*, Centre for Sexual Health Research, Faculty of Social Sciences, University of Southampton, 1998

105   R Ingham and G van Zessen, From cultural contexts to interactional competencies: A European Comparative study. Paper presented at AIDS in Europe, Social and Behavioural Dimensions, 1998

106   K Wellings et al, op cit, 1994

107   Health Education Authority (HEA) analysis of Health Education Monitoring Survey, 1995 and 1996

108   Health Education Authority, *Today's Young Adults: 16–19 year olds look at diet, alcohol, smoking, drugs and sexual behaviour*, London, HEA, 1992

109   J Coleman, Puberty: is it happening earlier? *Young Minds Magazine*, 34, 1997

110   S Prendergast, op cit, 1992

111   Mizz survey reported in the Guardian, 10/2/1999

112   Health Education Authority analysis of Health Education Monitoring Survey, 1995 and 1996

113   ONS analysis of birth and abortion statistics series, 1997

114   K Wellings et al, op cit, 1994

115   Health Education Authority, *Unintended teenage conceptions; Qualitative research to inform the national programme to reduce the rate of unintended teenage conceptions*, HEA, 1998

116   Health Education Authority/BMRB *Sexual Health Matters Survey*, 1998

117   K Wellings et al, op cit, 1996

118   S Cheesebrough et al, op cit, 1999

119   R Ingham and G van Gessen op cit, 1998

120   Alan Guttmacher Institute, Facts in Brief, 1998

121   Alan Guttmacher Institute, ibid, 1998

122   Public Health Laboratory Service (PHLS) Data from PHLS Communicable Disease Centre, 1999

123   PHLS, ibid, 1999

124   PHLS, ibid, 1999

125   PHLS, ibid, 1999

126   K Wellings et al, op cit, 1994

127   Wareham et al, Contraceptive use among teenagers seeking abortion – a survey from Grampian, *British Journal of Family Planning*, 1994

128   Family Planning Association, *Children who have children*, FPA, 1993

129   Department of Health annual return KT31 and Common Information Core

130   S Clements, N Stone, I Diamond, R Ingham, Modelling the spatial distribution of teenage conception rates within Wessex, *The British Journal of Family Planning* 24:61–71, 1998

131   VAH Pearson et al, Family Planning Services in Devon, UK: awareness, experience and attitudes of pregnant teenagers, *British Journal of Family Planning* 21, 1995, 45–49

132   K Wellings et al, op cit, 1994

133   R Ingham and G van Gessen, op cit, 1998

134   J Brooks-Gunn and FF Furstenburg, Adolescent Sexual Behaviour, *American Psychologist* 44:249:257

135   G Duncan et al, Termination of pregnancy: lessons for prevention, *British Journal of Family Planning*, 15, 1990 p112–17

136   S J Brook and C Smith, Do combined oral contraceptive users know how to take their pill correctly? *British Journal of Family Planning*, 17, 1991 p18–20

137   P Donovan, op cit, 1998

138   The 1999 Durex Report *Spotlight on sex and sexual attitudes in '90s Britain*, Durex, 1999

139 HEA/ONS, op cit, 1998

140 G Duncan et al, op cit, 1990

141 Health Education Authority, *Unintended teenage conceptions, Qualitative research to inform the national programme to reduce the rate of unintended teenage conceptions*, HEA, 1998

142 M Simms et al, op cit, 1984

143 I Allen et al, op cit, 1998

144 ChildLine response to the Social Exclusion Unit's consultation on teenage parenthood, 1998

145 I Allen, et al, op cit, 1998

146 K A Moore, B C Miller, B W Sugland, D R Morrison, D A Glei and C Blumenthal, Adolescent Sexual Behaviour, *Pregnancy and Parenthood: A review of research and interventions*, Child Trends Inc., 1996

147 B C Miller and K A Moore, Adolescent Sexual Behaviour, Pregnancy and Parenting: Research through the 1980s, *J of Marriage and the Family* 52:1025–1044

148 M Resnick, R Blum, M Smith, J Bose, R Toogood, Characteristics of adolescents who parent or place for adoption. Unpublished, 1989

149 B Maughan and A Pickles, Adopted and illegitimate children growing up in L Robins and M Rutter (eds) iv *Straight and Devious Pathways from Childhood to Adulthood*. Cambridge. Cambridge University Press, 1990

150 R Winkler and M Keppel, *Relinquishing mothers in adoption*, Melbourn. Institute for Family Studies, 1984

151 ONS, Birth statistics series, 1998

152 ONS, ibid, 1998

153 ONS, analysis of abortion and birth statistics, 1998

154 ONS, Abortion Statistics Series, 1997

155 ONS, ibid, 1997

156 ONS, ibid, 1997

157 K A Moore et al, op cit, 1996

158 K Foster et al, op cit, 1997

159 K Foster et al, ibid, 1997

160 Social Exclusion Unit, *School Exclusion and Truancy*, The Stationery Office, 1998

161 Department for Education and Employment, Social Inclusion: Pupil Support, Draft Guidance 1999

162 J Corlyon and C McGuire, *Pregnancy and Parenthood, National Children's Bureau*, 1999

163 J Corlyon, ibid, 1999

164 K Kiernan, Lone parents, employment and outcomes for children, *International Journal of Law, Policy and the Family* 10, p 233–249, 1996

165 J Bradshaw et al, op cit, 1996

166 C Davies, A Downey and H Murphy, *School age mothers: Access to education*, London, Save the Children Fund 1996

167 L Burghes and H Brown, *Single lone mothers: Problems, prospects and policies*, Family Policy Studies Centre, 1995

168 I Allen et al, op cit, 1998

169 HEA analysis of data on living arrangements from surveys on smoking and pregnancy, 1994–1998

170 I Allen, et al, op cit, 1998

171 K Kiernan, op cit, 1995

172 B Botting et al, op cit, 1998

173 S Speak, et al, op cit, 1995

174 I Allen, op cit, 1998

175 D Birch, *Young Fathers,* paper presented at an International Conference on Adolescent Health. Youth Support, Royal College of Physicians, London, 1998

176 K Kiernan et al, op cit, 1998

177 J Wilson, op cit, 1995

178   K Wellings et al, op cit, 1996

179   S Meadows and N Dawson, *Teenage mothers and their children: factors affecting their health and development*, 1999

180   S Peckham, op cit, 1993

181   S Speak, S Cameron and R Gilroy, *Young single fathers: participation in fatherhood – barriers and bridges*, Family Policy Studies Centre, 1997

182   M Mauthner and V Hey, Case study of teenage parenthood in a London Borough for the Social Exclusion Unit, 1998

183   National Foster Care Association – *Foster Care in Crisis*, NFCA, 1997

184   Department for Education and Employment, *Preparing Young People for Adult Life*. A report by the National Advisory Group on Personal, Social and Health Education, 1999

185   Department of Health Consultation Paper, *New arrangements for 16 and 17 year olds living in and leaving care*, forthcoming summer 1999

ANNEX 10: CONSULTATION

The Government would welcome views on how local co-ordination can be improved to meet the target given in this report.

Specific issues you might focus on are:

■ What are the most important things that need to happen to make sure that the local strategies work, and what are the risks?

■ How can local co-ordinators best be supported?

■ How can the range of organisations that need to be involved (including local authorities, health authorities and voluntary organisations) best be engaged?

■ Is there additional work that needs to be undertaken at the national level to help the strategy succeed?

Please send your answers to these issues and other related questions to Mandy Jacklin at Department of Health, Wellington House, 135–155 Waterloo Road, London SE1 8UG by **30 September 1999**.

Please say if you wish your response to be treated as confidential.

Printed in the UK for The Stationery Office on behalf of the
Controller of Her Majesty's Stationery Office
Dd.5068839, 6/99, 5673, Job No. 81911